CRITICAL ACCLAIM FOR
An Uncertain Inheritance

"These essays about caring for gravely ill parents, partners, even children, meet a real need. . . . Though wrenching, the stories provide solace and practical advice." —*People*

"Honest. . . . [A] remarkably wide spectrum of experiences is covered." —*New York Times Book Review*

"A godsend for many readers." —*Newsday*

"The essays in editor Nell Casey's *An Uncertain Inheritance* are revelatory glimpses into the everyday agonies and occasional flashes of rapture that caregivers experience." —*Vanity Fair*

"In these achingly powerful, expertly written accounts, we are given rare, invaluable glimpses into an unavoidable aspect of being human." —*Elle*

"A remarkable array of mostly original essays by talented writers on being cared for themselves and caring for parents, children, and spouses with illnesses as varied as depression and brain injury. . . . Well worth reading." —*Publishers Weekly*

"Each essay explores the burdens, terrors, sorrows, and, occasionally, joy involved in undergoing a terrible ordeal with someone you love. . . . A beautifully written but painful series of meditations." —*Kirkus Reviews*

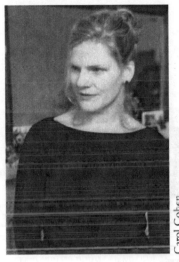

About the Editor

NELL CASEY is the editor of *Unholy Ghost*. Her work has appeared in *Elle, Mirabella*, the *New York Times Book Review*, and on Salon.com. She is a Carter Center mental health journalism fellow, and is on the board of Stories at the Moth, a nonprofit storytelling organization. She lives in New York City.

ALSO BY NELL CASEY

Unholy Ghost: Writers on Depression

an uncertain inheritance

WRITERS ON CARING FOR FAMILY

EDITED BY NELL CASEY

FOREWORD BY FRANK McCOURT

HARPER PERENNIAL

NEW YORK ● LONDON ● TORONTO ● SYDNEY ● NEW DELHI ● AUCKLAND

HARPER PERENNIAL

FIRST HARPER PERENNIAL EDITION PUBLISHED 2008.

Designed by Gretchen Achilles

Library of Congress Cataloging-in-Publication Data has been
applied for.

ISBN 978-0-06-087531-2

08 09 10 11 12 ID/RRD 10 9 8 7 6 5 4 3 2 1

contents

FRANK MCCOURT   *Foreword*   ix

NELL CASEY   *Introduction*   xiii

HELEN SCHULMAN   *My Father the Garbage Head*   1

SAM LIPSYTE   *The Gift*   12

ANN HARLEMAN   *My Other Husband*   19

JEROME GROOPMAN   *Elliott*   34

JULIA ALVAREZ   *Caring Across Borders: Aging Parents in Another Country*   66

STEPHEN YADZINSKI   *Called Them Vitamins*   77

JUSTINE PICARDIE   *Ruth*   88

ANDREW SOLOMON   *Notes on Accepting Care*   94

ANNE LANDSMAN   *The Baby*   102

ELEANOR COONEY   *Death in Slow Motion*   118

ED BOK LEE   *Mourning in Altaic*   146

SUSAN LEHMAN   *Don't Worry. It's Not an Emergency.*   164

ANN HOOD   *In the Land of Little Girls*   175

AMANDA FORTINI   *The Vital Role*   188

SCOT SEA   *Planet Autism*   208

ABIGAIL THOMAS   *The Day the World Split Open*   219

STAN MACK   *The Elephant in the Room*   228

KERREL MCKAY   *Transformed by a Touch*   245

JULIA GLASS   *The Animal Game; or, How I
                  Learned to Take Care of Myself
                  by Letting Others Care for Me*   252

                  Contributors   271

                  Acknowledgments   279

                  Permissions   281

foreword

The telegram was addressed to someone at "The Hospice for the Dying." I suppose I should have felt a chill when I looked at that envelope and realized I'd be delivering that telegram.

Instead, I felt merely curious. The hospice was somewhere on the edge of my town, Limerick, and I wondered if I'd see anyone dying.

A man at the gate told me to go up to the front door and if I met anyone I was not to talk to them.

"Are you listening? Talk to nobody."

I promised I wouldn't say a word, but I rode my bike slowly in hopes of seeing dying people. There were some old men on benches chatting and smoking pipes, and they looked too lively to be dying.

A man answered my knock at the front door. Because this was a church institution, I knew there would be no tip. That freed me to ask, "Are those old men out there dying, sir?"

I thought he was going to hit me. "Get out of here, you little twerp, or I'll give you a good fong in your arse."

A few days later I had telegrams for the Limerick Lunatic Asylum, which sits strategically next to the Limerick Jail, beyond which is the St. Lawrence Cemetery. Beside the jail there was a pub and, across the street, a hospital.

All very convenient.

Eventually, there were telegrams for the jail, but I was unable to see the prisoners. I climbed a wall to see if there were any "lunatics" walking around the yard of the asylum, and I was delighted when some spotted me perched up there and threatened to come up and tear the head off my shoulders and shove it up the hole of my arse.

I had a great time sitting up there on the wall, taunting them, and an even better time telling my family about the experience. My brothers laughed, but my mother took me aside and told me those poor people were special to God and anyone who laughed at them was laughing at God. She said I should go around the corner to the church and tell St. Dymphna, patron saint of lunatics, how sorry I was.

When I read the book you have in your hand, memories like these flooded back. I thought of a cousin of my mother's who sank into a depression, wouldn't move from the fireplace, refused food, and was forcibly taken to the lunatic asylum. His wife protested. She said a man shouldn't be put in the asylum for being sad. The men in the white coats said they had no time for her and her caterwauling.

A few weeks ago I attended the funeral of William Styron in Martha's Vineyard. I'm sure everyone in that little cemetery thought of the horror of his episodic descents into depression and how he made that depression public in a small but remarkable book, *Darkness Visible*. It was no secret that his depression paralleled that of Mike Wallace and Art Buchwald, all brilliant, remarkable men.

I keep digressing here—from what I don't know. This is the effect this book might have on you. It leads you back into your own life, where you are sure to find some aspect of yourself.

There are, I think, two great themes in this book: suffering and heroism. Here is a line from Steve Yadzinski: "No one's personality is suited to the transformation from health to sickness."

You're right, Steve. Unless you grow up with the chronically ill or surrounded by dying elders, you are simply not prepared for deterioration, decay, death itself. We *know* our parents will age and die, but when it happens, it's a shock. Helen Schulman writes, "My father started dying twenty years before he died."

Shock? You'll be shocked by the honesty erupting in some of these narratives, the mixed feelings we have when our parents—or family members in general—suddenly become so much of a burden we have to change our lives, move to other places, start the death watch.

Read this book slowly and discover nuggets of wisdom. Julia Alvarez quotes a popular Dominican saying: "The devil knows more because he is old than because he is the devil."

At the end, after the heartbreak and the humor, the dignity and the grace of these "caregivers," you'll want to stand and cheer.

FRANK McCOURT

JANUARY 17, 2007

introduction

NELL CASEY

Caring for someone through illness is an epic task. It requires such nimble fortitude—the ability to walk a tightrope of emotion as life hurries on indifferently around you—that it is hard to believe that the relationship is as commonplace as it is. In the United States, there are nearly thirty million informal caregivers[1]—defined, in the study *Economic Value of Informal Caregiving* by Peter S. Arno, Carol Levine, and Margaret M. Memmott, as people who provide unpaid help to relatives or friends with an illness or disability that leaves them unable to do things for themselves.

I have been a caregiver myself. I saw my sister, Maud, through a five-month depression, which occurred after she'd been hospitalized for a manic episode. It was a devastating experience. And yet, looking back, my story practically sings with triumph when I consider how it might've gone, how it so often goes. Maud was not on an irreversible downward slide—it was possible for her to get better—so, for all of us, there was an end in sight. And a happy one, as it turned out: Once Maud got back on her feet, she returned to her life with tenacity and success. My family, meanwhile, was given the pleasure and satisfaction of believing that our hard work had paid off, that we had helped Maud.

Seeing a family member through a health crisis is an experience that nearly everyone must face—even if it's only to make arrangements for someone else to do it. And yet caregiving, as a rite of passage, is only just beginning to enter our cultural and literary consciousness. (In part, this may be because, in describing the act of tending to the ill, language can veer into clinical descriptions—terms like "toileting" and "assisted living" come to mind.) There *are* excellent narratives in which caring for family is the theme—Ted Hughes's collection of poems *Birthday Letters*, *The Story of My Father* by Sue Miller, Lorrie Moore's short story "The People Like That Are the Only People Here," Philip Roth's *Patrimony*, and *The Year of Magical Thinking* by Joan Didion, to name some of the very best. But together these have not created a literary genre all their own, sparking a national discussion about the broader dilemma, as with, for example, motherhood or depression.

Perhaps, as with death—so often a part of the caregiving experience—it is not something many of us want to look at directly. We'd prefer to take furtive glances, quietly fending it off until suddenly called upon by someone in our own family. And who can fault us for not wanting to spend more time in sorrow's grip? Still, seeing an intimate through illness is a meaningful pilgrimage, one that calls on us to know how much we can and will sacrifice for those we love.

And it is becoming increasingly necessary. The average life span is growing longer—it has extended by about four years for both sexes since 1980[2]—and, with the first wave of Baby Boomers already in their sixties, the need for care at the end of life is more dire. (Not to mention that, since many are choosing to become parents later, there are now approximately sixteen million Americans catering simultaneously to the needs of elderly parents and young children—the so-called Sandwich Generation.[3]) Only three years from now, by 2010, it is expected that the number of people age eighty-five or older in the United States will rise by more than two million.[4] Meanwhile, already an estimated 80 percent of all home care for the elderly—from giving baths to monitoring ventilators—is provided by family.[5]

This collection illustrates an experience that is in flux: Caregiving is a growing aspect of our society but we haven't yet paid adequate attention to it. By bringing many writers to bear on this subject, the hope is that everyone will find a story with relevance and value. These are predominantly stories of ailing mothers and fathers—reflecting the fact that nearly three quarters of caregivers look after an elderly parent—but some writers explore their bonds with afflicted husbands, wives, siblings, and children.

The opening essay, Helen Schulman's "My Father the Garbage Head," is a beautifully rendered criticism of the tendency to idealize the caregiver, to blithely and grandly suggest that people who choose to care for another will be rewarded for their efforts. Schulman also rails against her own mortal limits. "My love wasn't going to ease his pain, and it certainly wasn't going to save him," she writes about her father. "How could this be? I wondered. How could this endless reservoir of affection and attachment and respect that I felt for this man prove so powerless?"

And yet some do find, in more complex and precise form, a version of the reward that others promise for taking on this burden. "It's a different marriage from the one we started with," Ann Harleman says of her partnership with her husband, who suffers from multiple sclerosis. "A marriage I would have refused on that evening twenty-five years ago in the California garden where we first met. A marriage I could not have hoped for, or even imagined, in the dark days five years ago. . . . I am thankful that we found it in time."

A turning point often found in these narratives is the realization that no amount of devotion can fully lift the burden of another's pain. It is at this time that, to paraphrase Freud, acute misery becomes ordinary suffering. One must move past the early heroic rush and settle in for the long, earthbound haul. Some cross this threshold and maintain a sense of purpose; others don't.

"Moneylessness, my manuscript deadline, guilt, sorrow, relentless responsibility, and no life of our own: we were trapped," Eleanor Cooney writes of the consequences of bringing her Alzheimer's-afflicted mother to live with her and her partner, "swimming hopelessly in circles, sinking, hearing my mother's ever-narrowing set of refrains, recited daily like the stations of the cross, each one a knife in my heart." Cooney plainly—and poetically—describes the ways in which she was forced to lose her mother again and again and again.

And yet, even in some of the most unyielding narratives, there are moments of grace. "Once, lying on her bed," writes Sam Lipsyte about being with his dying mother, "talking, talking about nothing in particular, maybe something reported on CNN, maybe our old life in New Jersey, maybe something about her parents, because I'd begun to delve into the past with her, I studied her as hard as I could. Her eyes were closed, and for the first time I could actually sense the end of her, her body. And lying there beside her was so sweet. Why couldn't we just have done that *all the time?*"

Julia Glass, Andrew Solomon, and Amanda Fortini give voice to the other side: that of being cared *for*. In doing so, they reveal the helplessness of surrendering to another, the paradox of both wanting attention and not, and the emotions that rise up after the crisis has passed.

"What I didn't tell [my husband], but should have, was that he was doing something just by being ... with me," writes Glass of her battle with breast cancer (while also raising two very young sons). "I began to understand that taking care of someone doesn't always mean doing something for that person. . . . Being is just as important as doing. Being awake. Being present in the next chair. Being funny. Being smart in a surprising, useful way. Being sympathetically perplexed. Being a mirror for the expression of pain."

The enormous expectations inherent in this relationship, in addition to the beleaguered intimacy, can also bring anger and disappointment. "My father's kindness at some level reminded me of my own helplessness," Solomon admits. "He meant his assurances to be uplifting, but sometimes they felt like trivializations of my very real condition. I was not going to be fine and I wanted him to acknowledge that. I was indebted to him, but my appreciation teetered constantly at the brink of ingratitude."

"One of the most trying aspects of being sick is being cared for, as counterintuitive and thankless as that may sound," declares Fortini. "Nothing makes a person feel out of control—and illness by definition is a loss of control—like having to cede it to another person."

Tensions can also radiate outward, affecting others in the family. When her elderly mother and father moved back to the Dominican Republic, and began to struggle with their health, Julia Alvarez and her three sisters were thrust back into the competitive dynamic of their adolescence, vying for their parents' attention even as they were ministering to them. Anne Landsman also had to take into account her siblings in relation to her dying father. When Landsman decided *not* to go to her father at the end of his life—for complex reasons she explores in her essay—she quietly worried about the judgment of her brother and sister.

An acute feeling of self-consciousness is woven into many of these essays. "'How are you managing?' friends ask. 'How are you doing this?'" Abigail Thomas writes, describing the reaction to the news of her husband's traumatic brain injury after being hit by a car. "Doing what? I wonder. This is the path our lives have taken. A month ago I would have thought this life impossible. Sometimes I feel as if I'm trying to rescue a drowning man, and I only have time to rise to the surface for one gasp of air before I go back down again. There is an exhilaration to it, a high born only partly of exhaustion, and I find myself almost frighteningly alive"

These authors, granted an elemental wisdom from their suffering, lay bare the complexities, the unexpected compensations, and the private sadness of being relegated to this no-man's-land of illness. These are honest narratives, sometimes with a sense of optimism, sometimes not, but where the writers don't offer hope, they offer companionship. They've been there, too. And so, it is from this "unfamiliar country," this other "planet," within this "black balloon"—as the landscape is variously described throughout—that these contributors offer their soaring missives.

Finally, this truth emerges: We endure.

1. Arno, Peter S., "Economic Value of Informal Caregiving," presented at the Care Coordination and the Caregiving Forum, Department of Veterans Affairs, NIH, Bethesda, MD, January 25–27, 2006.
2. National Center for Health Statistics, Department of Health and Human Services Web site, www.cdc.gov/nchs/.
3. Kuba, Cheryl, *Navigating the Journey of Aging Parents.* New York: Brunner-Routledge, 2006.
4. United States Census Bureau.
5. U.S. General Accounting Office, "Long-Term Care: Diverse, Growing Population Includes Millions of Americans of All Ages," 1994.

an uncertain inheritance

my father the garbage head

HELEN SCHULMAN

My father started dying twenty years before he actually died. He had a heart attack and bypass surgery while I was still in college. From that point on, although my mother had three different cancers in the intervening years and a host of other medical problems, it was the specter of my father's death that floated above us at all times, perhaps because he himself feared it so. He was an atheist; he was terrified of his own nothingness, the inevitable empty void that he could not rationalize away. And for years, as his child, my father's death was the thing I too was most afraid of—until it wasn't anymore, until the quality of his life, his unfathomable suffering became the most frighteningly real of nightmares and then I had more pressing things to be afraid of, like that he might, against all odds, continue to live.

The last ten years of my father's life were hard. The last five were horrific. It was during this long final phase, when his many illnesses became acute—swirling around in his body like some toxic murky stew, leaving him virtually paralyzed and as mindless as any late-stage Alzheimer patient—that I vowed to stay by his side, to help take care of him as long as he needed. I was married by then. I had first one, then two small children, a household to run, a career to manage, but my father had always stood by me, he'd loved me and cared for me my whole life, and in turn, I loved him without reservation. So I made a pledge.

"I will help him as long as he needs it."

I remember the moment I said this to myself outside his hospital-room door. It was a promise I lived to regret.

In the sexy, wild seventies, when I was a teenager, if anyone were to hold out a handful of assorted pills in the schoolyard of my high school and some kid was eager to randomly pop them, that kid was called a "garbage head." No drug of choice, just a messy indiscriminate addiction to all of it. During the last years of his life, my father—physician, professor, chief of two medical departments—was what I always thought of as a neurological garbage head, not just because he downed a hodgepodge of pills daily, but because he was afflicted with so many diseases that I pictured his brain itself as a myriad array of garbage. People would ask me what was wrong with him and I didn't know exactly how to answer them. What was right with him? He had coronary artery disease, had had numerous ministrokes (TIAs) and several larger ones. Until his autopsy, which concluded that he died of advanced arteriosclerosis, we thought he had Parkinson's; when he still could walk, he took those little mincing steps that Tim Conway made famous on the old *Carol Burnett Show*.

Five years before his death and about a week before the birth of my second child, my little boy, my father had one of those many strokes followed by an angioplasty and ended up in the same hospital where I was scheduled to give birth, the same hospital where he had practiced medicine for forty years.

"Hey, Dad, maybe I could take that bed over there and we could share a room," I teased, "and then you could stop stealing all of the attention."

Truth be told, I wouldn't have minded sharing a room with my father. I'd never had enough time with him—he worked endlessly when I was a kid, he was preoccupied with his own inner life, and while we were very close, he had a more natural affinity for my brother. Still, I always liked to be with him. Even after he was hopelessly brain-damaged I would often lie down on the bed next to him, in the hospital or at home in front of the television, and hold his hand.

So back then, when he'd only had his second real stroke—the "salad days," I call them now—I suggested sharing a room with my dad, but he didn't respond to me. He kept saying, "It's like I'm two, it's like I'm two," because, in the salad days, he still had the cognitive powers to know exactly what bad shape he was in: that he had the reasoning capabilities of a toddler.

On the phone a few weeks prior, when my father was bemoaning the collapsing state of his memory, I'd said, "I know that this is very hard for you, Dad, but we all love you, we still can have fun together, we still can enjoy one another, does any of that help at all?"

He said, "No, you and your love don't help me."

How his words stung me. At first they felt almost coldhearted, cruel. I was offering him the best of myself, but that seemed to mean nothing to him. My father was in many ways an insightful and responsive man, a generous man, but he also had this extraordinary allegiance to honesty; he could be candid to the point of insensitivity and at times, even selfishness. At the moment that he gave me his response, he was not thinking about my feelings, but rather solely about what he knew to be the truth about himself. My love wasn't going to ease his pain, and it certainly wasn't going to save him. How could this be? I wondered. How could this endless reservoir of affection and attachment and respect that I felt for this man prove so powerless, so worthless?

I did not believe him then, but I believe him now.

Ten days after that second stroke I was home with a newborn baby and a two-year-old daughter. A friend taught several of my classes for me, and then I went back to work, resuming my usual schedule of teaching and writing. Night after night I spoke to my parents on the phone. Consumed with worry, I called them every morning. There was reason to worry—my father would get stuck in the bathtub and my mother would have to call the doorman up to help her lift him naked and wet from the water. She'd feel dizzy or faint and find herself lying on the couch or the rug while he called helplessly for her from the other room. I ran across town to my parents' apartment on afternoons and evenings. My brother and I checked in with each other before every weekend, one of us taking Saturday to drop by, one of us taking Sunday. We were afraid to go away on vacation. We tried to convince my mother to get some help in the house. She didn't want help in the house. It was her house, her life.

The tipping point in my father's long descent came when he fell trying to get to the bathroom one night. The result of that fall was two massive cerebral hemorrhages and two brain surgeries. For a while there, he looked like a character out of *One Flew Over the Cuckoo's Nest*, with his shaved head, the twin tracks of staples in his scalp, his open mouth, his diaper.

For six weeks after my father fell I spent every day in the hospital. Sometimes I'd be there eight hours, ten hours, and when I left to return home to my own family, my mother said my father would open his eyes and say, "Why didn't Helen come today?" It was a black hole of time and energy, sitting by his bedside, willing him to wake up, screaming at the doctors, the nurses, the therapists, double-checking the medications because of course they were wrong—I don't know how many times they brought him penicillin when he was allergic to penicillin—begging for services, holding my father's helpless hand.

No one who cannot advocate for themselves should ever be left alone in a hospital. I remember once visiting my father in rehab. Someone had left the lunch tray in front of him. All he could do was stare at it; he couldn't negotiate the knife, the fork. They might as well have opted to starve him to death.

Those six weeks when he was mostly unconscious, I consoled myself by thinking that even if he didn't remember I was there, I *was* there, looking out for him. Perhaps some of our collective care, that of my mother and my brother and I, my estranged sister who visited sporadically, was seeping into his bones.

I took the semester off from teaching; I screwed up a writing assignment. My work and my pocketbook were suffering. My husband was kind, loving, supportive—a knight really—and I did my best to hold up my end at home, but it was hard on him, and the children felt it.

"Are you thinking about your father again?" my daughter asked me, when I stared off into space in the middle of reading her a story. "Don't think about him anymore."

Once he returned home several months later, my mother miraculously continued taking care of him, now with the help of several home health-care attendants. It would have been impossible otherwise, but she'd only allow help in the house during the day. She didn't want them in her apartment at night. She didn't want them on the weekend.

"You have to cook for them," said my mother.

"No you don't," I said.

"They are human beings. They need to eat," she said.

"Of course they need to eat," I said. "But you don't need to cook for them. You can pay them to buy the groceries. You can pay them to cook for you."

"Daddy wants me to take care of him," she said.

"You do take care of him," I said. "But you're going to destroy yourself and then what will happen to Daddy?"

"You have to talk to them, they have needs and problems," she said. My mother was a social worker. Soon her home health-care attendants were taking swimming lessons while they were on her time clock, they were studying for the GED. It was hard to argue with that kind of altruism, except that it increased my mother's burden, which in turn increased mine.

My brother and I would take her out for coffee. "You need more help," we'd say.

"Screw you," my mother said. She was angry at the world.

"You need to turn the house into a nursing home or you need to put him into a nursing home."

"It's my life," said my mother. But it was our lives, too.

She was exhausted and angry and doing her best. She schlepped him from physical therapy to cognitive therapy to museums to the movies, all of it a losing battle. At night she'd cry to us on the phone. My parents had had a true romance. They had talked and fought and had fun for forty-something years, but now, at times he even forgot who she was.

"Mom's driving me crazy," I said to my father. "She needs to take a break, go away for a weekend or something."

"Who's Mom?" he said.

"Gloria," I said.

"Who's Gloria?" he said.

"Your wife," I said. "My mother."

"My mother?" he said. It was like a vaudeville act. The Parkinson's-like symptoms had increased and his limbs became so stiff he could not move them; he was confined to a wheelchair, he could not inch himself over in bed. The fact that we later found out he didn't actually have

Parkinson's meant only that the Parkinson's medications we shoveled into him by the vial-full were useless.

At times, when he could talk—weeks went by, it seemed, without his talking, and then out of nowhere, a pair of sentences—he thought his own parents were still alive. It was like that movie *Groundhog Day,* we'd have to give him the bad news again and again: "Daddy, I'm so sorry to tell you this because I know you are feeling mixed-up today, but you are seventy-eight years old and your mother died thirty years ago." Each time his pain was fresh and raw, my comforting hand on his arm eventually produced by rote. At times he hallucinated. For a while, he thought bears were eating him—probably due to the medication we were giving him for the Parkinson's he didn't actually have.

Weeks and months would go by, we'd try to achieve a new normalcy, and then there would be another spiral downward. I'd bring the children to see my parents and when we'd near their building my son would run away: "There's sick people in there," he'd say. My mother would put my daughter on my father's lap, and he'd pee in his pants.

"Shhhh," I'd say to the children when they wanted me to play with them in the evenings, the phone receiver glued to my ear and chin, "I'm talking to Grandma."

I'd sit in a chair next to the bed and hold my father's hands, so thin and so cold. An old man's hands, gnarled and stiff as wood. They were my mother's husband's hands, the hands he used to hold her, to touch her. I forgave her everything, and I forgave her nothing.

"It's my life," my mother said. "Screw you."

My brother and I talked on the phone.

"He's killing her."

"She's killing me."

"We have to kill him."

"We can't kill him."

"We have to kill him."

"If you really think we have to kill him we shouldn't be talking on the phone."

We'd meet in a bar. "How can we kill him?"

It wasn't like we could withhold treatment or anything, he wasn't being kept alive, he was keeping himself alive—he and his fear of death, he and his iron will.

"Your mother takes too good care of him," said a doctor friend. "Put him in a nursing home, and he'll die in three weeks."

But is that what I wanted? My father to die in three weeks?

"Perseverance conquers all," read my father's motto in his high school yearbook. As a Jew (in a time when there were Jewish quotas) and a middling student, my father had applied to seventy-five medical schools before he got his first acceptance. He was trained for a year at a school that then lost its accreditation. He retook the same year at another institution that then lost *its* accreditation. He went on to Chicago Medical School and became president of his class. Chief resident at Mt. Sinai. His whole life had been about tenacity. But he couldn't conquer death, could he?

"My parents are killing me," I told my husband. "You'll see, I'll predecease them." I was being melodramatic, but I also wasn't. It had taken my husband and me years to have a family. This was supposed to be our time to enjoy it. We were at the last, tippy-toe edge of youth, and it was being squandered on hospitals and bedpans and exhaustion. The stress was enormous. I was offered an academic position, and my mother said, "Don't take that job, your children are only young once, and I may need you."

My brother and I met in another bar.

"It's agony watching him suffer."

"No one should live like that."

"We could use a pillow."

"We could go to jail."

"We could give him pills."

"That's murder."

"I don't want him to die."

"*He* doesn't want to die."

"He doesn't want to die."

"Well nobody does."

Nobody does. But there was simply no pleasure left in my father's life, he couldn't even smile when the kids came over. All he did was suffer.

And yet when he could talk, he'd say with fear in his voice, "Am I going to die?"

I called my mother: "This year, don't give Daddy a flu shot."

My life became an endless game of gambling on what I hoped would prove to be lesser evils, an endless practice of emotional triage. Should I stash the kids with the neighbor as I rushed to meet my parents in the emergency room? Should I accompany my critically ill mother in an ambulance and leave my father helpless and alone at home? Should we prosecute the home health-care attendant who wrote thousands of dollars of checks to herself from my father's checkbook? But would that leave her pregnant teenage daughter without financial support?

All that tender loving filial care was supposed to help my father, but it didn't. It was supposed to build me into a better person; make me more compassionate, effective, stronger. I think that people like to believe there is a reward in the end for caregiving. There were no rewards. There was only my father's compelling need, and my useless love for him.

After my father died, the subject of my own death came up in a therapy session. I was with my father when he died, and I didn't want my own children to have to bear the burden of that. I didn't want my husband there, either. Everything good in my life has radiated from my husband, why should I put him through a scene that he would never get out of his head? It was not the way I wanted him to remember me.

"So you want to die alone?" the shrink asked. I thought *Yes I do, I want to die alone.* There are many, many things I prefer to do alone. Then I thought, *No, it might be too scary all alone,* so I said in one of those ludicrous pronouncements you make on the shrink's couch, "I figured out who I want to be with me when I die." (As if one could choreograph such a thing.) "My father. I want my father there."

"But he's dead," said the shrink, being a shrink.

"He can come back," I said. "He owes me."

But of course who owed whom and what? I owed my father my life. The piano and the ballet lessons. The camps and vacations and the fact that

I did not have to work my way through college even though he thought
it was a waste of time to want to be a writer. When I was a kid, we used
to sit some nights together on the big green chair in our living room and
have talks. "What do you want to talk about tonight?" my father would
ask. "Books," I'd say. I always said books. He wasn't a big reader, my father,
but he tried. I think that was what I appreciated most about him, what
glued me to him long after sense and reason told me to cut bait, to drive
my own car with its own set of needy passengers and leave him behind.

"Eskimos have it right," I'd joke bitterly when people would inquire
after his health, as if I ever could have possibly sent him out on his own
ice floe. He wasn't the strongest man on earth, he was sensitive and preoccupied and he openly struggled to rise to the demands of his days—but
he always cared and he always tried and he never gave up, not on anything
or anyone. I never saw my father give up on anything. After his brain surgeries, when he woke up out of his coma and saw my mother weeping in
the chair next to his bed, the first thing my father said was, "Gloria, how
can I help you?"

Later, when he was back home, my brother was leaving their apartment one day, and asked, "What can I do for you, Dad?"

In a rare moment of lucidity, my father said, "Have a good life."

The day my father died was my son's half-birthday. We'd been on
a deathbed vigil for three days and part of me just didn't believe he'd
ever let go. I was heading downtown to pick up the cupcakes my kid
loves—we cut them in half on half birthdays and then gobble both halves
up—when I decided to check in at the apartment for the second time that
morning. "You better come quick," said the home health-care attendant.
"He's going." So I called my brother and then I hopped into a cab and
raced across town.

The hospice nurse was there when I arrived, along with two attendants. My mother was sitting in the chair next to my parents' bed. They
were all watching my father breathe, loud laborious breaths, drowning
breaths as he fought the fluid flooding his lungs. There was blood on the
pillow; apparently he had hemorrhaged and been washed and cleaned
several times since I had been there the day before. My mother had been

up all night with him. She had been by his side the last three days. She'd always been by his side. Now she sat exhaustedly weeping in the chair, brokenhearted. I sat down on the bed.

"Dad, I'm here. It's Helen, Dad. Mom's here, Gloria, your wife is here." I said this because I didn't know if he could hear me or not, in his loud, rasping coma; or, if he *could* hear me, whether or not he would know who she or I was. I said, "Dad, we love you. Gloria and I . . . It's Helen, Dad, your daughter, Gloria and I and Charlie, we love you. The kids love you. We all love you. You've been a wonderful father, Dad. A wonderful husband. A terrific doctor. A wonderful son. Everybody loves you."

I patted his arms, his trunk, his chest; I kissed his cold hands, his waxy face. I kept touching him, hoping the stroking would be reassuring as his chest heaved and he struggled loudly for breath. I was worried, so worried, was I doing something wrong? Was I the one he wanted there at that moment? It was so intimate. I kissed him again and again. "You've had a beautiful life, Daddy. Don't be afraid, we love you. Everybody loves you. We're here and we love you. Take it easy. Take it easy." I said "take it easy" because his breathing was so difficult, he was struggling so. I said "take it easy" because that is always what he said to me when I was upset or sad or crying. I stroked and kissed my father. "Take it easy, take it easy." The rest of the room disappeared. It was the same force of concentration I'd felt twice before in my life—when I was giving birth to a baby. Everything, I was focused in on everything he was.

"We love you, Daddy. Take it easy. You've had a beautiful life." When was he going to die? I thought, *When are you going to die already?* Because that breathing was something awful. I thought, *Open your eyes, cut this out! Sit up and talk!* Because none of it felt real, and yet his heart was still beating and he was right next to me and the trunk of his body was warm and there I was, kissing and holding my father. "Take it easy. Don't be afraid."

Finally, finally, his breathing slowed, and agonizing gasp after agonizing gasp it slowly stopped, and then his eyes rolled up into the back of his head. My mother said, "I never saw anyone die before," and I turned from him to her and we hugged and cried and comforted each other. I said, "I think Daddy's dead. May I close his eyes?" She nodded yes, and so with two fingers I closed my father's eyes. We were both crying then, and hugging and talking. There was a strange, weird energy in the room, like when you've finished a race or exams are over. You're all charged up with nowhere to go, and yet you're completely spent.

Five minutes must have gone by and then out of nowhere, we heard him take a huge breath. My father, not dead, my father breathing, and we were back by his side.

He took another heartrending breath and then another, and his eyes opened, and I was back to my vigil, kissing and stroking, "We love you, Daddy, everybody loves you." I wanted to kill myself for closing his eyes before. Did he know? Did it scare him? Was he angry with me? "We love you, Daddy." In my arms with his eyes open his whole body began to shake and I could hear his voice, my father's doctor's voice, ever curious and instructive, the scientist in him speaking. I heard him speaking in my own head, and he said, "That's the death rattle." And in my own head, I said back to him, "Wow, so that's what it's like. I've read about that before."

Then his body stopped shaking and his eyes turned upward, and suddenly a huge cannonball of hot white light shot up from my pelvis through my body, my neck, and my face and out the top of my head— that's exactly what it felt like. As it passed through my head I could even see the flash of the light as it rocketed behind my eyes. And then my heart started beating wildly and now it was my whole body that began to shake and I broke out into a cold sweat, rivulets of water running down my legs, my arms, my spine. This must be adrenaline, I thought, in the moment, although later when I confided the experience to Charlie, he said, "It must have been his life force." Whatever, it was like a cannonball of light that shot through my body out of the top of my head, and if felt like there was a giant exit wound at the top of my skull, like my brain and all my interior were open to the air. I was shaking and I was crying. It was a terrible ending to a tortured life. No matter all that endless outpouring of my useless, useless love. His skin was already turning blue, his body was as empty as a shell you'd find on the beach, his nose looked like the beak of a fossilized bird.

He was so dead. He was so gone. And I no longer had a father.

the gift

SAM LIPSYTE

When a friend told me my mother was giving me a gift, my first instinct was to belt the guy. It's a good thing I've never belted anybody. Still, what kind of gift is the chance to stand around helplessly while your mother dies? I chalked up my friend's comment to one man's attempt at pseudospiritual spin. He meant well.

Secretly, I sensed he might have a point, too, though maybe not the one he intended. You see, I was the perfect caregiver: broke, needy, damaged, sad, hoping to avoid staring too long at the wreck I'd made of my life. It was good to have something else to stare at.

I'd wrecked my life with a lot of bad drugs and bad decisions made in the interest of the bad drugs, and now I was back home in my mother's apartment, twenty-four years old, a ridiculous cliché of self-infliction.

My mother, who'd spent more than twenty years as *my* caregiver, let me stay rent-free while I "cleaned up my act" and got a job. This I did. It wasn't a very polished act, but it *was* clean; and it wasn't any kind of fancy job, but it let me pitch in a little for food—or at least my food.

Though the prospect scared the hell out of me, I was beginning to imagine getting out into the world again, trying to be a functioning human. Then one day my mother told me and my sister, who was already a functioning human, that her breast cancer, in remission for thirteen years, had recurred. I wondered who was going to ease my mother through this awful time while I was out in the world rebuilding my humanity. I was sort of relieved when I realized it was going to be me. Why knock yourself out trying to resuscitate your life when you can cling to somebody else's?

That's a pretty severe way to view it all, I guess, but I've always been wary of this topic. It runs the risk of too much self-congratulation. You can dwell on your failings or marinate in muddied motivations, but, finally, you are pounding your chest, saying, "At least I was there."

I was there, and I wasn't there.

There had been sickness in my family before. My father had testicular cancer when I was ten, my mother her first round of breast cancer a few years later. Though my sister and I were in proximity to the horror show, we were mostly sheltered from it. We'd get a bucket for our puking father, wonder at this mysterious disease that made him weak and patch-haired, but the more serious problem we faced was how to convince our mother to buy us some Count Chocula.

So despite our family's long association with the medical-industrial complex, I didn't really experience it until my mother got sick again. There were lots of tests and lots of consultations. There were drugs and new drugs. There were occasions when I, the former needle man, got to employ the skill set of my old habit by injecting my mother with various injectables. (I tended to make a grand, nearly cinematic deal of flicking the bubbles away, as though to say, "Now, Mom, aren't you glad I was a junkie?") There were counts to count. There were agonies to monitor. There was the growing unspoken feeling that all the drug injecting and counting and monitoring wasn't doing much good; my mother was dying no matter what.

When I think of my mother's body, I think of a body in crisis. I remember her telling me how I'd been a cesarean birth. (The cutting out of her first child, a stillborn, necessitated in those days the same mode of entry for subsequent progeny.) She loved to quote the line in *Macbeth* about Macduff being "untimely ripped" from his mother's womb. As a kid I used to draw pictures of myself as a newborn, ripped from my mother's womb. Maybe that was weird.

Weirder is my earliest memory, my mother sitting in our living room with some friends. The afternoon sun is coming through the bay windows, and she is radiant in a dark, low-cut dress; I feel the most wonderful little-boy-in-sudden-view-of-his-mother feeling well up in me. I bolt across the room to embrace her, and just as I'm about to throw my arms around her neck, I vomit all over her breasts. Now it's a crisis. A shower needs to be taken. Somebody needs to watch me while the shower is taken. But the crisis subsides. She comes back fifteen minutes later, fresh and wet and radiant in another dress.

I'm not sure why this incident sticks with me, but it does. Maybe it's because my mother was not the most serene person, but when things got uncomfortable, or threatening, she grew steadier. Cancer summoned forth in her a grace and humor that she could never find for bad parking spots or botched restaurant orders. Suffice it to say that against current pop wisdom, she sweated the small stuff. But I think it helped her cope with the big scary stuff that always seemed around the corner.

My mother had a mastectomy after her first go-round, a radical mastectomy, and the term, in my adolescent mind, was somehow infused with a sense of danger and excitement, like radical politics. Sometimes my mother wore a prosthetic in her brassiere, sometimes she didn't. Once, when I was about sixteen, she asked if I wanted to see the scar. I didn't, but said yes, because I figured only a jerk would say no.

I still believe that.

After my father left her, my mother tried dating. It was hard going for a woman in her late fifties and eventually she had some reconstructive surgery. Whereas she'd had one large breast now she had two tiny ones. They even made a nipple from some other skin, colored it red. I'm not sure any of it helped that much.

When she got sick again, and I was her sidekick, I tried to at least appear to be the conscientious caregiver, the dutiful son. It was important to me, because I'd been a distant, possibly shitty, at the very least annoying and disappointing, son. I was her fallen golden boy and here was my chance to atone. I'm not sure if it occurred to me that I was mostly concentrating on appearing dutiful, rather than being so, but after a while they blurred together. If you want to be seen as somebody who has done the dishes, the shopping, the laundry, cleaned the house, organized the pills, your best bet is to actually *do* those things. I'd tote the notebook for our meetings with doctors, and eventually I started taking notes.

My father always said you had to "charm" doctors into caring about you. You are auditioning for a part in the doctor's psyche. Otherwise you're just meat. I don't think he's wrong. Often I wondered how the audition was going. I'd try to gauge the effect my mother—a smart and talkative woman who could be quite funny and blunt but also could babble on too long—was having on the busy, distracted doctor. I wondered if I was part of this audition, too. I recalled that scene in the movie *Fame,* where the girl tries out for the Performing Arts High School but it's her dance part-ner, Leroy, the judges get excited about. What if my "talent" was acciden-tally discovered just by sitting there? What if some compelling calamity was suddenly revealed in me? Of course, this was just a coming attraction. After a parent dies, not so deep in your thoughts is this notion: I'm next.

I don't remember all the bus rides, the cab rides, the hospital visits, the home chores and duties. Sometimes it all looms symbolically in my mind as a mighty ziggurat of Ensure cans. Or really I do remember all of those things, but not like I remember my moments of weakness, my failures of character. One night my mother was hobbling around the living room, weeping, moaning. I just wanted to watch some stupid television show. I told her to stop being so dramatic. The next day at the hospital we discov-ered the cancer had eaten through a good part of her hip.

Another time, I'd gone back to the apartment of a woman I knew. It was maybe the only date I went on during this period. We were fooling around. But I wasn't really enjoying it. It wasn't her fault, but I felt this in-tense fear. I just didn't want to face a moment of intimacy. Flesh-on-flesh was too much. I stood and started to dress.

"Where are you going?" she said.

"Look, I have to get out of here," I said.

"What's wrong?"

"What's wrong? My mother has cancer!"

Whenever I told people what I was doing with my life, living at home, helping my mother during her illness, they'd give me that sweet look, the one that made me cringe. Or else I'd get a story about how good it was I was there because so-and-so wasn't there and never forgave himself.

"Shit," I wanted to say, "I forgive him."

Until she got too weak to do really anything at all, my mother kept working on her novel. She'd published one in the mid-1970s, and she'd been working on the second ever since. There had been many iterations, many detours and wrong turns. Her old agent and editor had deserted her, or at least that's how I heard it. She struggled for years. She was stubborn. I honor that stubbornness by dragging around the boxes filled with all the versions of her novel from apartment to apartment. I haven't read them yet. I don't know when I will. But I will drag the boxes from apartment to apartment. Until I stop doing so. But for now there is something nearly corporeal about having all her manuscripts with me. I'm not much of an urn guy.

We watched a lot of television. We could have been reading each other poetry, I guess, or at least classic novels, but we filled our heads with garbage. Maybe the stink of garbage warded off the stink of death. Or maybe we were just pretty tired.

Once, lying on her bed, talking, talking about nothing in particular, maybe something reported on CNN, maybe our old life in New Jersey, maybe something about her parents, because I'd begun to delve into the past with her, I studied her as hard as I could. Her eyes were closed, and for the first time I could actually sense the end of her, her body. And lying there beside her was so sweet. Why couldn't we just have done that *all the time*? Why did we wait until the end to let go of everything that ever kept us from just lying there and talking like two people who are going to die and not be able to talk anymore?

Toward the end my mother was in and out of the hospital for weeks at a time. A few days into her last visit she called me from her hospital room. I'd been with her the night before and was planning to come back after work—I'd gotten a part-time job at an online magazine.

"You better come in now," she said. She sounded incredibly frightened, all her tough bluster blasted away. I called my sister, and we both rushed over. There were strange new machines in the room. My mother had suffered some kind of infarction. The doctor pulled us into the hallway.

"Your mother is going to die in a few hours," she said. "If you have anything to say to her, say it now."

My mother was manic. Her body was shutting down, but her brain was running crazily with morphine and adrenaline. The doctors were going to induce a coma. We were entering a "palliative mode." But for the next few hours, my mother kept talking. She told us she had no regrets, though I didn't really believe it. She asked for ice cream, but when we brought it to her she didn't seem interested anymore. We had a conversation about my new job. She was dismissive, said it didn't sound like much of a job. We bickered. We bickered in a way we'd often bickered, and I was horrified our last conversation, after all we'd been through, was a stupid spat. But now I see how fitting it was. She'd been the person who believed in me, or at least claimed to, even when by all external evidence I wasn't much more than a pathetic fuckup. That's the person you bicker with, even unto death. (Or at least that's what I tell myself.)

She didn't give up on herself, either. The few hours she was supposed to live turned into a week. We all gathered around her bed and ate Chinese food and told stories and lousy jokes. She was in a deep sleep, breathing on a ventilator.

Something happened during this time. I seldom talk about it, because it is implausible and sentimental and I sound like one of those nurses spouting crap about angels (there were a lot of them) when I relate it. It's one of those things that would get written out of a script because it's too sappy. But life doesn't always have a good bullshit detector.

So here it is: One night a friend and I were sitting with my mother. Everybody else had gone home for a rest and the room was quiet except for the deep, phlegmy thrum of my mother's breathing. (Cleaning out the weird gruel that bubbled up into her oxygen mask had become a part of our vigil.) The friend asked me some questions about my mother's past, and I launched into a very long narrative, basically the entire story of my mother's life as I knew it, from her early childhood in Depression-era Pittsburgh to her younger years in New York City in the early 1960s to her time making a family and discovering herself as a writer and feminist in New Jersey. I ended with her divorce and her return to Manhattan. I touched on as many of her travels and experiences as I could recall. Finally, at the close of my little biography, somewhat patronizingly, I leaned down and kissed my mother's hand and said, "I love you." Whereupon the ventilator seemed to stutter and my mother started to lift her head a little, straining from her pillow. She made this great wheezing sound through her mask. "I love you, too," she said, before collapsing back into her coma.

A creepy part of me still thinks I got that little bonus because I was there for her. (Give the golden boy his gold star, please.) But I wasn't the only one. My sister was a great help to her throughout this time. Even my father, my mother's ex-husband, came around. And I still berate myself for not being there more, not physically but psychologically, all those occasions I couldn't take it and I'd tune her out, retreat into something meaningless, erect some wall between her suffering and me. But I did this when she was well, too, when her suffering was the suffering of life, not death.

I guess that's part of being a highly flawed and functional human.

So what does all this get me, gift-wise? Some kind of wisdom or peace? I'm not sure about that. Sickness and death are still the terrifying and unknowable things they've always been. Still, when I'm not getting overanxious about the future or too remorseful about the past, I can cherish a few moments in the here and now with my wife, my son, my friends, my work. So, sure, it's a gift, but who wants a gift like this? What's worse, there is no return policy. I'd trade in any peace and wisdom for more years of bickering with my mother. But, sadly, the best you can hope for is that someday you get the chance to pass this gift on.

my other husband

I n the summer of 1980, the second summer we knew each other, we drove from Providence (where Bruce lived) to Seattle (where I lived). Somewhere in the middle of Montana, we hit a thunderstorm. I told Bruce how my little sister and I used to run around our backyard naked in the rain. How we loved the feeling of slickness, of intrusion, the warm rain alive on our skin. Bruce turned onto a narrow dirt road and stopped the car. He got out and walked around it into a little stretch of woods and began to strip. His shoulders, always unexpectedly beautiful to me, emerged round and smooth and shiny with rain. Rain glinted in his beard and the curly dark hair on his chest and belly and around his cock, which pointed toward me. When all his clothes lay on the pine needles around his bare feet, he stood there and looked at me gravely.

What could I do but get out of the car and take off my own? What could we do but make love?

AUTUMN 1999

I put my elbows on my knees and let my forehead sink onto my palms. I'm tired. Not just tired—weary. My husband's catheter went AWOL at one in the morning, and we've spent the rest of the night in the ER. (How many nights does that make, now? How many hours? The EMTs who came with the ambulance greeted me by name. "Where's Bruce?" they said, already on the stairs to our bedroom, with the stretcher between them.) Noise and cold and too bright lights and too bright student doctors. Repeating Bruce's history, over and over. Concussion; stitches; bruising; subdural hematoma; second concussion; hairline fracture; three different kinds of pneumonia. My husband in pain, and nothing I can do about it.

I must have slept, because suddenly Dr. Zayas is standing across the gurney with Bruce's hand between both of his. Bruce's eyes sweep over him with fevery incomprehension and keep moving until they find my face. I try to smile.

"Go home, Ann," Zayas says, his Russian accent hollowing out the words. "Rest," he says, his eyes full of compassion. They've replaced Bruce's catheter, but in the process they discovered another UTI, and the congestion in his lungs suggests pneumonia. He's been admitted; they're getting a bed ready for him. Zayas will call me later.

I kiss Bruce—his lips are alarmingly hot—and squeeze his toes in farewell, the way I always do, and slip through the heavy canvas curtain into the hall. One of the ER nurses gives me a plastic bag with Bruce's things in it.

By the time I leave, a cautious October sun reddens the sky above the parking lot, where the cold falls like a blessing on my hospital-hot face and birds measure out morning sounds in the trees overhead. At home I take the plastic bag of Bruce's clothes to the basement to put them in the washer. When I undo the string around its neck, the stench of urine nearly knocks me down. Holding my breath, pulling things out of the bag, I find everything—faded blue work shirt, khakis, boxers printed with little black keys—in pieces. They had to cut the clothes off him.

I make coffee, then call the university in Malmö, Sweden—it's midafternoon there—to tell them not to meet my plane tomorrow, the lecture and readings will have to be canceled, I am very sorry. I call our daughter, Sarah, who is just getting her boys up for breakfast. "Don't worry!" we tell each other, in unison. Brendan, Sarah's four-year-old, gets on to tell me they've just gotten a trampoline. I can come and jump on it, anytime. "Dzump!" two-year-old Timmy shouts in the background. "Dzump!"

Then, although it's only five-thirty A.M. in Chicago, I call my cousin Janet. When I hear her sleepy hello, I burst into tears.

. . .

In the days that follow, the house feels very empty. I should be glad of the time and peace, to work. I'm behind with deadlines—a book review, an article, corrections on the galleys for a story—and we need the money, because of the lost lecture fee from the Swedes. But I miss Bruce. I find myself with one ear out, the way you do with a child in the house. Listening for the sounds of him: the slap of the seat coming down on the stair lift, the hum of the motor as it glides down each flight, the thump that means he's made it safely into his wheelchair.

People—my friends, our families—seem to think of MS as something terrible that happened, once: a plane fell out of the sky onto our house. (This actually *did* happen to someone we knew: a small two-seater plane crashed into his house on a remote New Hampshire mountainside.) No. MS is something that goes on happening—growing, changing, worsening—measurable not in weeks, months, or even years, but in decades. Something huge and black that descends slowly and inexorably and surrounds you. More like a dirigible. Bruce and I have christened it the Black Balloon. To anyone who sees me—friends, family, students, strangers at my readings or lectures—I seem to be in their world, the world of the well. Going about my work, going about my life. But actually, I am inside the Black Balloon with Bruce.

In the bathroom, say, assembling the paraphernalia for his shot. (Somehow, no matter how careful I am with things—IV shunt, catheter, hypodermic—I always hurt him.) Kneeling beside his wheelchair, breathing in his familiar smell: baby powder, urine, and something less definable, the remote, forest odor of decay. *Okay.* Choose today's spot (there's a complicated rotation system involving arms, thighs, and belly), swab spot, insert fresh needle into holder, suck in sterile water 1.3 milliliters, inject water into ampule, turn ampule upside down until contents mix, suck in contents 1.3 milliliters (no air bubbles! flick with fingernail to disperse), hold needle poised in one hand, pinch husband's flesh between thumb and forefinger of other. The needle glitters in the lamplight. I plunge it in. Bruce winces. *Touch him. Give him his body back.* Slowly I draw the palm of my hand across his shoulders, under his woolen shirt. The skin feels warm and grainy. His eyes close in pleasure like a cat's.

Bedtime is when I feel his absence most. I miss things you'd think would be unmissable. Hoisting him up, coaxing the resistant flesh together; the weight of him, wheelchair to grab bars to commode to bed, thudding onto my shoulders and traveling down my spine; the separate sigh from each of us when at last he lies, more or less straight, in the bed; the cool gust from the down quilt as it settles over him; the snap of the bedside light, extinguished.

He loved my midriff. That was the word he used: midriff. It became a special word between the two of us, a courtly, Victorian code word for desire. He liked me to lie on top of the bedspread with my hair spread out around my head like (he said) gold wire and my back arched so that he could trace my ribs with his warm fingers.

Dr. Zayas calls. Bruce has been moved to intensive care. Earlier this afternoon there was a point where he stopped breathing, completely. They had to resuscitate him. He does have pneumonia, aspiration pneumonia—a bad one this time. He's on a ventilator. They need my permission to operate, to insert a feeding tube directly into his stomach so that he can't aspirate minute particles into his lungs anymore.

"He won't eat or drink at all?" I swallow. "Ever?"

"No," Zayas says. Emotion makes his accent stronger. "I am sorry, but not."

Bruce lies at a slant on the high bed under a stiff hospital sheet that leaves his feet bare. Corrugated plastic tubing, like a pastel vacuum-cleaner hose, protrudes from his mouth and snakes its way to a monitor on a metal pole. I stand at his head, the edge of the bed pressing into my pelvis, and look down. The ventilator's clear plastic mask flattens his beard and mustache; his face is pale. As if in response to the sheer force of my attention, his eyelids begin to flutter. *Open!* I say silently. *Open, now!* But they don't. Folding my arms for warmth—*Why is the ICU always so cold?*—I stand listening to the rhythmic suck and sigh of the ventilator.

After a few minutes Dr. Zayas appears in the doorway and beckons to me. I pull the sheet over Bruce's feet, which, as my hand brushes them, feel like stone. Then I follow Zayas down the hall to the intensive-care waiting room. We settle into slippery vinyl chairs between two family groups, one speaking fast, twangy Chinese, the other chattering in Spanish. The Spanish speakers throw us a few pitying glances—because we are so obviously not a family?—and Dr. Zayas, leaning forward, lays a hand on my arm.

He clears his throat. It's going to be The Conversation, again.

Quickly I head him off. "I've signed the permission form. Can someone here show me what to do? How the feeding tube works? For when he comes home."

A pause. Then Zayas segues into the familiar litany.

Skilled nursing.

Not safe.

Cognitive impairment.

Round-the-clock care.

"The G-tube—it is tricky. More tricky than the catheter. Things go wrong."

Bruce already refers to himself as Ports-of-Call, because of all the "ports"—permanent holes in his flesh—that admit various kinds of plastic tubing into his body. One in his groin, for the supra-pubic catheter; one in the back of his hand, for the IV that delivers steroids; one in the crook of his elbow, for the IV that delivers antibiotics. And now there will be one in his abdomen. His *midriff.*

"Also"—Zayas pursues his theme—"he needs a wheelchair all the time now. This he does not truly accept. Next time he decides he can walk, and he falls, he could break his pelvis."

"Bruce needs a blanket," I say. "A *couple* of blankets. It's cold in his room."

Zayas's dark eyes shine with sadness. "I wish I could offer you more," he says.

Sarah appears on the threshold of the waiting room with her sons. They know all about tubes—and wheelchairs, gurneys, IV poles, heart monitors. When he's older, Brendan may remember seeing Gramps walk; Timmy won't. The boys run across the room and throw themselves on me, fighting for my lap. Two beautiful boys, one tall and dark-eyed, the other compact and fair. I look over their heads at the Hispanic group.

See? I *do* have a family.

"You have lucky eyes and a high heart."

The first thing Bruce ever said to me, that June night twenty-five years ago. We were summer fellows at the Huntington Library in California, an impossibly beautiful place. The Reader Services librarian arranged a ride to the annual director's party for me. (An English professor at Brown, you have a lot in common, she'd said that afternoon. He'll pick you up at seven. He's a wonderful man.)

Tall; intent brown eyes under wayward eyebrows; curly, Old Testament beard. We introduced ourselves, shook hands. Behind us, in the faculty club's lantern-lit garden, a wedding reception was taking place. The orchestra finished tuning up and swung into "String of Pearls."

Bruce was still holding my hand. "Dance with me."

"But—we're not invited."

"Dance with me."

Impossibly romantic; but then, we were impossible. Tenured at universities three thousand miles apart. Impossibly older (him). Impossibly married (me).

When I was growing up in the 1950s, Catholics were discouraged—at least in my parish—from reading the New Testament by themselves. (You were supposed to get it in installments at Sunday Mass, pre-interpreted for you by Father Sawyers.) Of course this made it irresistible. My favorite story was the one where Jesus visits Lazarus and his two sisters. Mary sits at Jesus' feet, listening to him hold forth, while Martha bustles around serving, bringing food, cleaning up. When Martha complains about this inequity, Jesus says to her—I still remember the exact words—"Martha, Martha, thou art anxious and troubled about many things; and yet only one thing is needful. Mary has chosen the best part, and it will not be taken away from her."

In my family, "workhorse" was a term of praise. The New Testament gave me permission to be something else. I started small, with guerilla tactics. Go off to the woods for the day with my bike basket full of books instead of looking after my trouble-prone sister; pretend to need a lot of sleep so I could lie in bed under the eaves and daydream; develop allergies to dust, laundry soap, and the pigs' hairs used as bristles in scrubbing brushes. Gradually I expanded my scope. I held onto Mary in the face of my first family-in-law's tight-lipped disapproval of my staying in college instead of working my husband's way through; their even tighter-lipped disapproval over my going to graduate school instead of getting pregnant; the head-shaking of my professors when I *did* get pregnant. I held onto Mary through working motherhood (unusual in those days and deeply suspect), accusations of home-wrecking, divorce, giving up tenure.

Then came MS. And I had no choice but to become Martha.

The evening air is full of unshed rain. I must be driving more slowly than I realize: headlights loom suddenly behind me, slew sideways, shoot past, loom again. Low, womanly hills give way to the clustered lights of the city.

At the hospital, Bruce is being transferred from wheelchair to bed. I can hear the pumping of the Hoyer lift as I walk down the hall. From the doorway I watch the canvas sling that holds his big, fetus-shaped body travel slowly through the air and lower him onto ironed white sheets. After the nurse a dreadlocked young black man I've never seen before— straightens his legs and props him up on the pillows, Bruce gives me an evil smile. I realize too late I shouldn't have let him see me see him.

"Visiting the *bedridden*?" he says. "How sweet."

If you don't stand up to him in these moods, he gets worse. "Sarcasm is the lowest form of irony," I say.

Twenty years ago, when the symptoms started—four years after we married, five years before we found out his diagnosis—he began to change. His wry humor turned mean. There was the time he spent a whole evening mocking our old friend Hans, who was going deaf, by making him repeat everything. There was the time he threw his cane at the brand-new visiting nurse who fumbled his IV. And there's the way he was—the way he *is*—with me. Because I take care of him, I'm implicated in his illness. I have blood on my hands (or snot, or piss, or shit).

"I can leave, if you'd rather," I tell him.

The nurse, embarrassed for me, busies himself picking up things off the floor, where Bruce has apparently thrown them—the moistened sponge-on-a-stick that he sucks now instead of drinking water, several crumpled Kleenex, the remote for the TV. He's not really like this, I want to say to the dreadlocked young man. I want to tell him about my Other Husband. The one who couldn't wait to kiss me when he came in the door every evening, who often kissed me right up the stairs into bed before he even took his coat off; the one who got up with our daughter when she had a bad dream and gave shadow plays on the wall by her bed until he made her laugh; the one who—

"So many flowers, you'd think I was dead," Bruce says.

It's true: on the windowsill are two enormous bouquets whose cards say, "Much love, Mom," and "Your loving bother." In these periodic crises, Bruce's stepmother and brother generally opt for phone calls or, one step further removed, FTD.

Bruce, watching me read the cards, says, "Bother, is right." And we both, to the surprise of the young nurse, start to laugh.

Crossing the parking lot in the rainy dark, I hear the cheery hello of Sylvia B., two notes, like a doorbell. Sylvia is president of the Well Spouse Organization. She's been visiting her husband, too—a handsome man with a cockatiel's crest of pure white hair, who was once a concert violinist. She's here all day, every day, feeding him (though the nurses would prefer to do that), reading to him, playing Chinese checkers (she moves the pieces for them both). She wears Chanel suits in beautiful muted tweed—she's around seventy, I think—with a colorful silk scarf looped around her throat over her pearls. Her shoes match the scarf. Her clothing tells you that these visits are her vocation.

"Oh, Ann!" she flutes. "How is Bruce? I looked in on him this morning, just to cheer him up a bit, but he was sleeping."

I'll bet he was. "Better," I say.

"You'll be taking him home soon, then. That's *wonderful!*"

We end our comrades-in-arms exchange with Sylvia recommending that I get a kneeling van, she doesn't know how she ever lived without one. I watch her walk away, her step jaunty.

An admirable wife. But I have seen her husband's trapped look as she pushes the spoon against his tightly closed lips, and her own lips curving in triumph when she wins.

In the fall of 1990, five years after Bruce had first begun to have serious symptoms, we'd been waiting a week for the results of the MRI. It was a hot, somber, dark-skied afternoon. Bruce took my hand and led me upstairs. We sat, not quite touching, on the edge of our bed while he told me.

Chronic progressive multiple sclerosis My first reaction was relief. There was a cause, after all, for the aching joints, the falling, the swift changes in mood. And the cause wasn't fatal.

I put my arms around him. He kissed me and kissed me, his mouth on my eyes and nose and chin, his beard scratching my cheeks.

"We won't let this affect our lives," he said.

And in my innocence—my utter, enviable ignorance—I nodded.

Chronic = always.

Progressive = worse and worse.

Multiple = many (all up and down the spinal cord, which Zayas calls
   the body's sine qua non, its marrow).

Sclerosis = hardening (as in, hearts).

My cousin Janet flies to Providence from Chicago for a long weekend. We sit, bundled in sweaters with quilts over our knees, in my dying garden. The late October sun polishes Janet's dark hair to a crow's-wing shine. Leaves litter the flagstones and lie in drifts along the high cedar fence.

"Bottom line," Janet says, "he's not safe. What's your plan?" She's seen me through my divorce, my parents' deaths, my sister's suicide. She's entitled to cut to the chase.

"I can take care of him," I say.

But Janet knows about the nurses I've hired to stay in the house when I've had to travel, fired by Bruce as soon as my plane took off; about the neighbors I've asked to look in on him, driven away by his angry outbursts; about the MedicAlert medallion that he throws in the wastebasket.

"You can't be in the house 24/7. His brain is blue cheese. One of these days—when he thinks, 'What am I, Professor Bruce Rosenberg, doing in a fucking wheelchair?'—he'll stand up and take off across the living room and break a hip. Then where'll you be? Where'll *he* be?"

What is this sudden obsession with broken hips?

"Have you been talking to Zayas?" I ask.

Janet leans forward. "With chronic illness, a lot of times the caregiver ends up dying first. Out of stress and exhaustion. I've seen it."

Janet is a psychiatric social worker. But other people have told me stories—Zayas, the women in my Well Spouse Support Group, the nurses. *Well Spouse Drops Dead,* is how I headline them. I can't deny that it's a relief now to drive homeward each evening with Bruce in safe hands. Not to pause, key in the lock, for that breath-held moment—*What will I find?* (Husband on the floor, blood pooling under his temple; husband sprawled headfirst down the steps to the basement; husband slumped against the kitchen cabinets, raising his hands to wipe off tears of fury.) But to make that relief permanent?

She put her husband away.

"There *are* good places," Janet says, reading my mind the way she has since we were kids. "I can tell you how to find one."

My eyes move over the leaf-strewn garden, the yellowed stalks of what used to be snapdragons, the tall skeletons of hollyhocks and sunflowers. "Fear no more the heat o' the sun," I murmur.

"What?"

"Shakespeare. It was the first thing Bruce said when they took him off the ventilator."

Janet stands up, sloughing leaves off her lap. "Who are you hanging onto him *for,* sweetie? Him—or you?"

. . .

That hot gray September afternoon fifteen years ago, after he told me, we made love.
Not desperately (that would come later). Not despairingly (that would come later
still). More like two people trying to say everything—past, present, future—in a
single telegram.

Afterward, we lay with our bodies tight together, our heads on the same pillow.
A hot breeze sifted through the open window. We could hear the far-off rumble of
a slowly approaching thunderstorm.

"Everything that grows," he whispered, in his Shakespeare voice, "holds in
perfection but a little moment."

AUTUMN 2005

Joanne, Bruce's favorite nurse at Tockwotton Home, greets me with a new
joke. "What was Helen Keller's favorite color?"

Behind her, in his battery-powered wheelchair, Bruce smirks. Clearly
she's already told him this one.

"I don't know. What?" I ask.

"Corduroy."

The three of us laugh. Joanne finishes pouring Bruce's ground-up
meds into his feeding tube, flushes it, hooks a fresh bag of liquid food at
the top of his IV pole.

"Chief nourisher . . . in . . . life's feast," he says. It's harder and harder to
understand him when he speaks; but somehow Joanne always does.

She shakes back her wild curly hair. "We'll hook you up when you're
back in bed, okay, Professor? See ya!"

He doesn't thank her as she leaves; he doesn't have to. Caring for his
traitorous body is her job—that's how they both see it. A job she does
with matter-of-fact grace.

I kiss Bruce, the familiar tickle of his beard and mustache like a separate wordless greeting. Very slowly he reaches up and lays a hand (his good
hand) along the side of my face. I settle into the chair beside him. "What's
new?"

He smiles. "New York. New . . . Jersey."

"New Mex . . . ico," we say in unison.

What can be new, when two people see each other every day, and one of them spends his day immobilized? We have our usual lopsided conversation, me recounting cute things Brendan and Timmy have said or done, describing what happened in class, passing on regards from friends. Bruce doesn't always follow what I'm saying; but it doesn't matter. We like being together. We like sitting side by side, striped with sunlight falling through the blinds of the west-facing window behind us.

I found Tockwotton by following Janet's instructions. Look for non-profit homes, she said—the staff are better-paid and therefore happier. Look for ones that have been around a long time. Small ones. Spend a morning in each place, don't say why you're there, just hang out. Use your eyes (How does the staff treat patients?), use your ears (How do they talk to them?), use your nose (Is the place clean? Are the patients? Does the food smell appetizing?). Make sure that when your retirement savings are used up and Bruce has to go on Medicaid, they'll keep him.

Now, almost five years since he first came to Tockwotton, Bruce is still in the same sunny room with its view of Providence harbor, surrounded by his favorite prints and paintings, bookshelves full of his favorite videos, plants, photographs of his wife and children and grandchildren. On one wall are the jackets of the twelve scholarly books he wrote, laminated and framed. His television is the best one at Tockwotton: when the Red Sox play, the staff gather in Bruce's room to watch the game, even though he's a Yankees fan. He has a computer that he uses every day, one-handed, incredibly slow, incredibly patient.

We sit in silence for a while. Then Bruce says, "There . . . *is* . . . something."

"Something wrong?"

"Something . . . new." He gestures toward the pile of papers beside his computer—old mail, monthly activity calendars, magazines he can no longer read but likes to save. On top of the stack is a painting on a sheet of stiff, heavy paper, composed of thousands of closely spaced stabs of color. Blues and mauves and greens: forested mountain slopes converge

and greet each other beneath a cloud-kissed sky. Looking at it, I am filled
with slow-blooming peace.

"A present?" I say, looking up. He's a favorite with the staff—men
are scarce in nursing homes, as are patients who can carry on a conversation—and they often give him things.

He smiles his old smile, the one that spreads upward till his eyes crin-
kle at the corners with the old wryness. He pauses, for dramatic effect.
Then he says, "Yes. For . . . you."

"For me?" Then I get it. "*You* did this?"

An art therapist came and gave a class, I find out later from Lisa, the
social worker. Each of the patients chose a page from a calendar and cop-
ied it. Bruce, who'd never painted a picture in his life, painted this one
with his left hand, brushstroke by brushstroke, over eight weeks. He'd
sworn the staff to secrecy so that he could surprise me.

"The acci . . . dental . . . artist," he says.

"It's beautiful." I place the painting carefully in my book bag. "Thank
you, sweetie."

All that labor, hour after slow, patient hour. But it isn't the labor he
wants me to admire; it's the painting itself. In this place I am Mary, not
Martha. Bruce is sometimes mean or sarcastic with the nurses or the
CPNs, but never, now, with me. Because I'm no longer his physical caregiver, I'm no longer implicated in his illness. His resentment of his body,
his despair over his inability to command it, his shame—these no longer
extend to me. Because our bodies don't connect, our hearts can. In the
time we spend together now we elude, for the moment at least, the bleak-
est premise of chronic illness: that one's body is one's fate.

It's a different marriage from the one we started with. A marriage I
would have refused on that evening twenty-five years ago in the California garden where we first met. A marriage I could not have hoped for, or
even imagined, in the dark days five years ago. I think of it as my Other
Marriage. And as I kiss Bruce good-bye and squeeze his toes and leave, I
am thankful that we found it in time.

· · ·

Now I can see that going into the nursing home not only saved Bruce's life but his spirit. And not only his but mine. At the time, though, there was no promise of this, or even hope of it.

There was the terrible aloneness of making the decision. I kept picking up the phone to call someone and talk it over, then realizing the person I wanted to talk to was Bruce.

There was emptying the house, dismantling twenty years of a life together. The day and a half I spent weeping while I unscrewed grab bars all over the house, feeling each room release Bruce and go slack.

There was the hunger strike Bruce went on his first day at Tockwotton, disconnecting his feeding tube and refusing to talk to anyone, even me.

There were the nights in my bare new apartment when I slept with the phone on the other pillow, so that I could meet Bruce in the ER whenever he had a crisis. And the nights when I didn't sleep at all, wondering what on earth I had done.

Timmy and I are jumping on the trampoline in his backyard, under the trees. The leaves of the maples, fiery red and yellow, catch and hold the late afternoon sun. It's warm enough—Indian summer, still—that we pull off our sweaters and throw them onto the grass below. Timmy's compact, blue-jeaned body rises and falls, his face pink with pleasure. I feel strong, soaring, invincible. Bounding; landing; bounding again. The sensation of being free yet impelled, in motion without effort—it's got to be the next best thing to flying.

"Nana!" Timmy says, between bounds.

"What, Gorgeous?"

"Gramps can't ever jump with us."

"No," I say. "He can't."

"Because his wheelchair would be too heavy."

He executes a perfect cannonball, then throws back his head and laughs. We jump facing each other, in opposite motion like a seesaw. I'm getting winded, but I don't want to stop. Timmy lands on his behind alongside me. Sunlight splashes his upturned face.

"Sweet!" he says. "The sky is bouncing, too."

I look up. A few soft-looking, pure white clouds have nosed in from the west. The sky above us is a mottled, imperfect, heart-stopping blue, like the sky in Bruce's painting.

"No, it's just us," I say. But Timmy is unconvinced.

"It could be," he says. "It *could.*"

elliott

JEROME GROOPMAN

J erry, it's Elliott. In Jerusalem. I know it's early, but it's an emergency."

Emergency. I felt a burst of adrenaline race through my body.

It was still dark in the bedroom. The glowing red digits of the night table clock read 5:03 A.M., making it just after noon in Jerusalem.

"What is it, Ell? How I can help?"

I imagined the worst—Elliott's wife, Susan, or son, Benjamin, injured by a terrorist bomb or a car accident.

"I have a growth of lymph nodes in my chest. It's interfering with my breathing. A few hours ago, my doctor told me I need surgery. What do I do?"

Elliott was transformed in my mind from one of my closest and oldest friends into a "patient." I mentally organized his particulars into the format of a clinical case: a forty-three-year-old previously healthy Caucasian male, non-smoker, working as a journalist in the Middle East, with enlarged lymph nodes in his chest, considered for surgery.

"Ell, tell me first what happened, from the beginning," I evenly replied, following the principle that the best history of an illness is elicited in the patient's own words. That way, the physician does not prejudice the recounting and keeps an open mind to the full breadth of possible diagnoses.

He had first become aware of something wrong eight weeks before, during his regular early-morning jog on the hills between West and East Jerusalem. It was a temperate spring day, the sun hardly over the horizon, the cool nighttime air from the Judean desert still lingering over the city. Elliott started at his house in the German Colony, at his usual pace, aiming to complete his regular four-mile course. But at the very first ascent, at Yemin Moshe, where the quaint Montefiore windmill stood, he had been forced to stop.

"My chest felt tight, heavy, like there was a weight pressing on it. I couldn't get enough air to make it up the hill. I figured I was coming down with a cold, and walked back home."

I asked Elliott if he had had any fever or chills. None whatsoever; he had checked his temperature when he returned from the aborted run, and several times since. Cough or sputum? He had recently developed a dry cough, but without phlegm.

As I listened, I was creating a list of diagnoses in my mind. By my own convention, I always started with the worst category. In the case of a mass of lymph nodes in the chest, it would be cancer.

I considered the different types. First, cancer of the lung: Elliott had never smoked cigarettes that I could recall. But lung cancer also occurred from exposure to environmental toxins like asbestos, once commonly used in house insulation. I recalled that Elliott and Susan had renovated their house in Jerusalem three years before. Elliott could have been exposed to the material then, but the incubation period from exposure to lung cancer was usually much longer, a decade or more. Next was malignant lymphoma: very possible, and often involving the chest. Lymphoma was classified as Hodgkin's or non-Hodgkin's types, and either generally occurred in teenagers and young adults when centered in the chest. I moved down the list to the less common cancers. Thymoma or cancer of the thymus gland: often associated with a disease called myasthenia gravis, which impairs muscle function. Elliott would not be regularly running four miles if he had myasthenia. Thyroid cancer: more frequent in women, and related to radiation exposure. Such exposure was remote for Elliott in his occupation as a writer. Testicular cancer: often overlooked and important to consider, since the embryonic testes originate in the upper chest and migrate during fetal development into the pelvis; vestigial deposits in the thorax can become cancerous in adulthood.

"Ell, you never smoked, correct? And you weren't in contact with asbestos during the house renovation?"

"Never smoked, except grass, of course. A contractor did the renovation, and we were assured for Benjamin's sake that all precautions were taken when they stripped the old pipes."

I continued down my mental list to the second category, infection. Tuberculosis: quite possible in a world traveler now residing in the Middle East. Fungal diseases like coccidioidomycosis: prevalent in the Sacramento Valley of California, where Susan's parents lived and Elliott often visited. Toxoplasmosis: a parasitic infestation from cats, ubiquitous animals, but generally causing a self-limited flulike illness. All three—TB, fungus, and toxoplasmosis—would have fever as a prominent manifestation, and Elliott had affirmed he had had a normal temperature throughout.

I ended my list with the category "miscellaneous," considering rare disorders like sarcoidosis. Sarcoidosis is a condition where the body becomes allergic to its own tissues, resulting in inflamed masses of lymph nodes in the chest. It is most common in blacks. There is scarring of the lung tissue which would be evident on chest X-rays in addition to the nodes. Sarcoidosis often caused red nodules in the skin and inflammation of the eyes.

"Any rashes or skin bumps? Do you have conjunctivitis or a gritty feeling in your eyes?"

"None of that, Jerry. I'm just totally winded. And not only when I try to run. Even walking fast I feel the tightness."

Elliott had begun to worry when the chest tightness persisted through the week. He called his general practitioner, Jeremy Levy. But the doctor, also an American who had emigrated to Israel, was on holiday out of the country. The covering physician had Elliott come to the office, but there he was not examined, not even his chest, just handed a prescription for erythromycin for a presumed bronchitis.

"Even though you had no fever or sputum?"

"Correct."

After two weeks on the antibiotic there was no change in his symptoms. His regular doctor was still away. This time the covering physician listened to his lungs and heard some wheezing. Elliott was told he might have asthma and was prescribed an inhaler. This afforded some relief, but he still couldn't make it up the hill when he tried to jog again.

"Finally Dr. Levy returned from the States. He ordered a chest X-ray. After two months of this growing inside me."

I maintained my calm and even voice, though I felt angry and anxious. My friend, a reliable person complaining for two months of a disabling symptom, had been incompetently evaluated. Critical time may have been wasted. For a fleeting moment I saw my father, gasping in the throes of heart failure, a general practitioner standing confused at his bedside. My father's life was lost because of medical mistakes. This memory painfully gripped me, and I forced myself to disengage from it and return my focus to Elliott.

"Did you have any blood tests? Did Dr. Levy describe what was seen on the chest X-ray?"

"I'm not anemic and my white count is okay. Susan had me get a copy of the X-ray report. It says, and I'm translating from Hebrew, so give me a minute: 'Enlarged mediastinal lymph nodes . . .' What's mediastinal?"

"Just medical jargon for the central area of the chest under the sternum, the breastbone."

"Right. 'Enlarged mediastinal lymph nodes measuring 8 centimeters in maximum diameter and surrounding'—better English would be 'encasing'—'the trachea and extending to the aorta. Compression of the right bronchus. Lung fields otherwise clear.'"

I paused to assess the information. The dimensions of the mass, the compression of his airway, and the adjacent surrounding unscarred lung, taken with the absence of fever or sputum, made cancer overwhelmingly likely.

I began to review my diagnostic list of cancers but felt my concentration slipping. It was not the early hour and interrupted sleep. Rather, my focus was clouded by a collage of intersecting memories—Elliott and I lingering over coffee in his Manhattan apartment, talking about his aspirations as a writer at *Time* and mine as a future doctor; Pam in her bridal gown and me in a tuxedo joined with Elliott in a triangular embrace at our wedding; Elliott gently dabbing drops of sweet red wine in my firstborn son Steven's mouth to "anesthetize" him before his ritual circumcision.

The collage was erased by the sound of Elliott's quivering plaintive voice.

"Jerry—what do I do?"

I paused a moment, then said: "Put Susan on the phone."

Susan, an émigré from California, worked as a political and business consultant and was a coolheaded master of logistics. Her native American optimism had been mixed with an acquired Israeli toughness, so in a notoriously bureaucratic country like Israel she was able to make things happen quickly and efficiently.

"Hi, Jerry," Susan began. "We really don't know where we are yet. I checked out the surgeon Dr. Levy recommended at Hadassah Hospital. He's said to be good. And I know enough powerful people there to make sure Elliott gets special attention. But we want the best, the *very best*, so maybe it makes sense to come back to the States."

The "very best" in clinical medicine was not only expert physicians and technologically advanced hospitals. There were many of those to choose from throughout the world. Serious illness demanded more. It was like a wild rodeo bronco, often exploding in unanticipated directions, stubbornly bucking to throw you off its back. The "very best" required tight and determined hands on the reins. There needed to be attention to every detail and nuance of diagnosis and treatment. Even seemingly minor errors—a misread CAT scan or a too rapidly administered medicine or the lack of an available catheter—could allow the situation to spiral out of control and be catastrophic. Who would exert such control in Elliott's case?

"I can't make the decision for Elliott and you. Medicine is quite good in Israel. You need to be sure that the specialist in charge will be totally focused on Elliott's case, covering every aspect of the situation. You also have to consider the practical dimension—your jobs, your insurance, Benjamin's school, and a host of other things holding you there."

Susan paused but a moment.

"But we don't have you, Jerry. We're coming to Boston. Expect us the day after tomorrow. I'll arrange to get seats on the next El Al flight."

It all happened in rapid succession. They arrived early Tuesday morning, just after my sons, Steven and Michael, left for school. Elliott was anxious and pensive, an ashen shell of his ebullient self. I embraced him forcefully, and could feel a weak shiver pass through his body as he tried to return my hug.

Susan quickly occupied herself with organizing their luggage in the upstairs playroom where Pam had opened the couch into a sofa bed. Benjamin, a cute three-year-old with jet black hair and almond brown eyes like his mother's, immediately fell asleep after the fifteen-hour plane trip.

Elliott and I sat in tense silence during the car ride to my office, each absorbed with his own thoughts of what the day would hold. I had designated myself as his physician of record and arranged for blood tests, a CAT scan of the chest, and appointments with Peter Draper, a thoracic surgeon, and Tom Cramer, an anesthesiologist, in anticipation of surgery the following day. Before sending Elliott off on this schedule, I thoroughly examined him.

I moved Elliott's long auburn hair off his neck so I could palpate for lymph nodes. He still affected a bohemian look, the same look he had when we first met two decades before. We had been introduced by a mutual friend, Anne Albright, who brought us together because she was struck by how similar we were.

"You could be brothers, so tall, with those deep-set, soulful eyes," Anne had teased us once over mugs of French roast coffee one Sunday morning in her Riverside Drive apartment.

But it was not just our physical resemblance that had struck Anne. She said it was how much we shared in spirit—our appetite for information, our sense of humor, our loquaciousness. Elliott and I had blushed at her bold praise.

"You look worried," Elliott stated as I removed my hand from his neck.

Just above his collarbone was a matted hard tongue of tissue. It resisted the compressive force of my fingertips. The mass was growing up now, from the mediastinum to the apex of his thorax. I had noted a subtle bulge in the veins in his neck, and a slowing of their rhythmic flow.

I hesitated in responding, not wanting to tell him what I observed. But I knew I should not deviate from my policy of honesty with a patient, even a patient who was like a brother to me, and whose condition caused me deep anguish. If I did not tell the truth always, I would not be trusted when I had a truth to tell.

I explained that the veins in his neck were dilated, and this indicated superior vena cava syndrome. The vena cava, the large vein that drains the blood from the head, was being compressed by the mass of nodes in his chest before it emptied into the right atrium of his heart. That backed up circulation in the brain and could cause increased intracranial pressure, manifesting first as a headache.

"I've had a constant headache over the last few days but figured it was stress."

I agreed that his headache could be due to stress, but the compression of the vena cava was contributing as well. By tomorrow we would diagnose the nature of the mass, and begin to treat it. That would decompress the vena cava.

Elliott looked knowingly into my eyes, and then returned my honesty with his own.

"Jerry, I think I'm going to die."

I shuddered at his words.

I had cared for many patients who had intuited their own deaths. Sometimes it was obvious to all, to patient, physician, family. Then the disease was widespread, the treatment failing. But occasionally there was no clinical sign that pointed in that final direction. I had come to believe strongly in how a patient feels and reads his body. Beyond any objective tests, blood chemistries, cardiograms, or CAT scans, a patient's sense of impending death often proved true.

I gripped Elliott's exposed shoulder tightly, holding fast, as I offered words of comfort. He was exhausted from the trip and from worry, I said, and should not rely on grim feelings in such a state. We did not yet know the cause of the enlarged lymph nodes. Once we made the diagnosis, we would embark on our course of action.

But as I continued with my reassurances, I studied the distant look in his eyes, and wondered whether he had indeed seen the arrival of life's last visitor.

· · ·

"Scalpel"—"Scalpel" ; "Clamp"— "Clamp" ; "Suture"—"Suture."

We were well into the second hour of the operation. Peter Draper, the thoracic surgeon, had finished dissecting between the vital structures of the mediastinum—heart, aorta, lungs—and had just reached a dense band of inflamed fibrous tissue overlying the mass of nodes.

I stood slightly away. It was too distressing to watch a person whom I understood as I understood myself—as thoughts and feelings projected in the external form of the body—exposed as a conglomeration of tissues and vessels seeping blood and lymph.

I looked upward from the operative field. Elliott's lids were closed over his china blue eyes, and his face rested in a motionless mask. He had been transformed by the anesthetic into that intermediate state between what we know as life and what we imagine as death, where consciousness and feeling are suspended. In this state, I pictured his soul waiting in the anteroom of time, ready to pass back into life should the surgery succeed, or exit on its voyage with death. As I gazed at Elliott's immobile form, I silently prayed for his return to life.

Elliott's life. I knew its intimate details, learned during twenty years of friendship.

He had been a child prodigy from an Orthodox Jewish family in Brooklyn, excelling in languages, mathematics, music. His father, whom I still deferentially referred to as Professor Ehrlich, was a renowned scholar of medieval Jewish history at City College; his mother was the principal of a Hebrew high school.

Elliott was the first student from his yeshiva to go to Harvard, where he graduated magna cum laude in American studies. Following in his family's professorial tradition, he began a doctoral program in colonial history at Yale. But he found the academic life too quiet and staid, the dimensions of the ivory tower too small.

So he left Yale for a job at *Time* in New York. For a while Elliott had found it exciting. It wasn't the New York he had known—Brooklyn with its sedate, tree-lined streets with two-family houses and elderly denizens chatting on the sidewalks. It was Manhattan, with all its intensity, grit, and ambition. At *Time* he found many like himself, educated at Ivy League colleges, poised to conquer the larger world. It was when Elliott was at

Time and I was a medical student at Columbia that Anne Albright introduced us.

Although Elliott had made a living at *Time,* what his parents called a "decent" living for a single person in Manhattan, after three years he felt unsatisfied. The thrill of seeing his name among several on a joint byline waned, and he did not advance to a regular national column or produce an article that was considered for a national prize.

In June 1976, as I was leaving New York for my internship in Boston, Elliott quit the magazine and set out for L.A. He hoped Hollywood would provide what Harvard and Yale and *Time* had not.

"You bring yourself wherever you go," his father reminded him. I recalled remarking to Elliott at the time that it was the kind of advice my father, had he been alive, would have offered.

I heard Peter Draper sharply announce that he had snared the upper lip of the mass and that the attending pathologist, Ned Waterman, should enter the operating theater. I watched Peter deliver a glistening cube of tissue from the deep cavity of Elliott's open chest. He placed it on a sterile gauze sponge and then cut it into three equal pieces. Ned Waterman quickly moved his pathologist's forceps onto the field and distributed each piece into a different receptacle: one flash frozen in liquid nitrogen; one placed in a plastic container with fixative; the last dispersed into a cell suspension in a saline-filled tube.

Peter Draper looked up and nodded to me. It was a signal that all was proceeding smoothly. I relaxed a bit, feeling the tension in my legs ease, and returned to my thoughts of Elliott.

Perhaps he occupied such a special place in my life because, among all my friends, he was my alter ego. Through his odyssey I acknowledged my own restlessness, my own fantasies of taking risks in life, of deviating from the path of the "good Jewish boy."

When I left Harvard for my training in hematology and oncology at UCLA, Elliott was working as a scriptwriter in Hollywood. He lived in a rundown cottage on a hill in Malibu, overlooking the churning Pacific Ocean. There, Elliott entertained glamorous women he met at the studios, charming them with his humor and warmth.

His quest was to write a film about the formation of the first-generation

American identity. He searched for cinematic venues not only in urban centers but in the far reaches of the country, traveling to the remote Arizona desert, small towns of east Texas, the wild chaparral of Montana. He sought inspiration as well in marijuana and tequila. As he reached more deeply into the diversity of American culture, he became ambivalent about his parochial background. Still profoundly bound up with the Jewish people, their triumphs and neuroses, he was nonetheless eager to stretch his roots—suspending his celebration of religious holidays, no longer keeping kosher, preferring the company of non-Jewish women.

Elliott was financially successful in L.A., earning a hundred thousand dollars or more a year on options for scripts. A few of his works became TV movies, and one was almost made into a motion picture but was killed at the last minute by the studio that bought it. The major project on the American experience—his serious work of cinematic art never came to be.

The surgical team was closing now. The ribs were realigned and the final sutures placed in the overlying skin. Elliott soon would be re-formed as he had always appeared to me.

In the adjacent room Ned Waterman, the pathologist, was already studying the slices of snap frozen tissue to obtain an initial diagnosis. I exited the operating room to join him. As I sat at the two-headed microscope with him, I began to review in my mind the diagnostic list I had formulated, but my thinking stalled. I felt my deeper mind repelling my conscious aim, as when two magnets are brought together at the same poles.

I suspended my effort to review the diagnostic list and momentarily retreated into recollections of the past, before the emergency phone call some four long days before.

Elliott stayed in L.A. after I came back to Boston. We spoke often, and I heard the disappointment in his voice as he described deal after deal that did not come to fruition. Three years after I left UCLA, in the summer of 1986, Elliott decided he needed a break from Hollywood. He traveled through Europe and then to Israel, where his parents had retired. At a garden party in Jerusalem, he met Susan. They fell in love, married, and Elliott started yet another life, in Israel.

Elliott told me how he looked forward to living in Jerusalem, how he imagined the city would be his teacher. He believed that the radical change in culture from the superficial, narcissistic world of Hollywood to the ancient holy city would nourish his creative powers and facilitate his writing of a major work. To support himself he took a job as a columnist for a new English-language periodical, the *Israel Bulletin,* and a position teaching film criticism at Hebrew University.

"Look at those cells," Ned Waterman said.

Gazing into the aperture, it was hard to comprehend that the tissue I was studying under the microscope was a part of Elliott. The magnified field should have been recognizable but was confusing, almost surreal. Large cells swirled and danced like the intoxicated moon and stars in the frenzied paintings of the mad Van Gogh.

"It's a T-cell lymphoma," Ned Waterman tersely concluded.

My heart sank.

I tried to sustain my emotional equilibrium and think about Elliott's situation in a considered clinical way. I recited to myself the details of T-cell lymphoma, as if I were teaching on rounds with a group of medical students and interns: *T-cell lymphoma represents some 2 percent of adult lymphomas. It is aggressive, marked by invasion of vital organs, particularly liver, bone, and brain. It is generally of unknown etiology, as it likely would be in this case. Recently, a mutation in a tumor suppressor gene called p16 was found in T-cell lymphoma. The p16 gene normally puts a brake on cell division in the T-cell, but when mutated the genetic brake loses its traction and the cells are released in a headlong rush of growth. There is a rare form of T-cell lymphoma endemic in southern Japan and the Caribbean. It arises not from a mutation in the p16 gene but from infection with a virus called HTLV, an acronym for human T-cell lymphoma/leukemia virus.*

I halted my didactic mental exercise, recalling that I had studied HTLV at UCLA in the late 1970s, while Elliott lived on the hill in Malibu. Could he have contracted this rare virus from one of his many romantic liaisons? We would test him, but it would almost certainly be negative.

I paused, my mouth dry, feeling slightly nauseated. I envisioned the next steps. We would clinically stage his lymphoma, assessing by CAT scan and tissue biopsy where, beyond his chest, the cancer cells might be growing. Although it might be confined to the mediastinum, given the size of the nodes and the two-month delay in diagnosis, I suspected we would find it elsewhere.

Elliott then would require very intensive treatment. At least five different chemotherapy drugs, administered together, for twelve months, followed by six months of so-called maintenance therapy with three more agents. The aim was to destroy every last lymphoma cell. The treatment likely would bring him to the cusp of death, damaging much healthy tissue—in bone marrow, liver, skin, mouth, and bowel—in order to purge the cancer completely.

My mind stumbled in its clinical mode as I considered the prognosis of a forty-three-year-old Caucasian male, previously healthy, with T-cell lymphoma presenting as an eight-centimeter chest mass. The numbers would not hold together. Each time I approached the statistics on long term survival, less than fifty-fifty, my heart sank again.

I knew at that moment that I could not be Elliott's doctor. For the first time in my career I had reached my limits as a treating physician. I was unable to function with the clinician's necessary analytical detachment. I realized that my inability was not just because of our closeness. It was that Elliott was too much a mirror of myself.

His situation had sparked memories of my father's death, of my youth as a student, and of my dreams as a physician-in-training. The arrival of Benjamin and Susan had made me consider how Pam would manage with our children if I were the one suddenly stricken with a life-threatening disease. In the operating room I had averted my eyes because I feared seeing myself as he was then, exposed for what we all are: vulnerable flesh and blood. Later, during his therapy, I would wonder how the poisonous drugs flowing into his veins would feel flowing into mine. And I shuddered at the thought. I knew I would perceive the final throes of his death as a vision of my own.

I realized I could not trust myself to be his primary care provider, to walk each morning into his hospital room and see the suffering that had to be if he had any chance of surviving—the vomiting and diarrhea and hair loss and bleeding and fevers and infections and mouth blisters and skin sloughing and a host of other side effects from the treatment. I feared that his physical suffering and psychological anguish would color my judgments and cause me to make a mistake—a mistake that could cost him his life.

I would never forgive myself for that, as I never forgave the physician who failed my father. That physician did not know his limits. I knew that my father might have died even in the most competent hands and the most modern hospital. But then I—and my family—would have known that all had been done that could have been done, and we would live without added anguish or regret.

I could think more clearly now that I understood the basis for my inner conflict.

I decided I could not, would not, remove myself entirely from Elliott's case and medically abandon him. I desperately wanted to help.

I arrived at a solution. I would offer myself as a "physician once removed." My scientific knowledge and technical expertise would be brought to bear at each step of Elliott's illness as they might be useful. After the clinical staging of the lymphoma, I would identify a competent and committed oncologist. With this specialist, I would help set the treatment strategy and advise on the medical response to problems and complications—as they undoubtedly would occur.

I stood in the surgical recovery room, grasping Elliott's pale hand. Susan leaned over him, wiping beads of perspiration from his forehead with a damp cool cloth. She took the news of his cancer without flinching. I sensed she had expected it from the start.

"Elliott will defeat it," Susan forcefully asserted. "I know him, how tough and determined he can be."

Elliott looked at her with measured appreciation. He whispered, his voice still heavy from the anesthesia, an echo of her sentiments: "I'm ready to fight. I want to live. Above all for you and Benjamin. And my daughter to be."

I looked at her with surprise, and then understood. Susan had seemed heavier, her taut facial features subtly expanded, her waist wide. I thought it was the first changes of middle age, she being in her early forties.

Susan smiled softly at me.

"I'm just in the first trimester."

"*Mazel tov*," I congratulated them, wishing literally "good luck." The traditional phrase hung heavily between us. We would need all the luck possible for their unborn daughter to know her father.

Later that evening in his hospital room, after Elliott had taken his first nourishment and the effects of the anesthetic waned, we began to discuss the logistics of his care. I began by outlining the further staging that needed to be done, two separate biopsies of his bone marrow and an MRI scan of his brain followed by a spinal tap. We would begin a short course of radiation to the mass tomorrow to free the vena cava and restore the free flow of blood from his head.

I hesitated and then, in faltering speech, began to discuss the question of where he should receive his eighteen months of chemotherapy.

Elliott looked knowingly at me. Before I could broach the issue of my being his primary physician, Elliott asserted that it didn't make sense to be treated in Boston. Now that the situation was under control, we could think more pragmatically.

He reached for my hand, gripping it with considerable force. He said he knew I would be there for him every step of the way, and my presence meant a great deal, more than he could express. But someone else, whom I knew and trusted, should take over his case.

I rallied, feeling grateful he had read my feelings and relieved me of my conflict.

We analyzed the options of which location and hospital and medical team would be the very best, and concluded Elliott should go to Alta Bates Summit Medical Center in Berkeley, California. A warmhearted and skilled colleague, Dr. Jim Fox, directed its outstanding program in blood diseases and cancer. Jim, I knew, would make the personal commitment to Elliott's care. A key factor in this choice was Susan's family. Her parents lived in Sacramento and owned a condominium in San Francisco. Susan and Benjamin would stay there while Elliott was receiving treatment. When the new baby arrived, there would be the support and resources of nearby grandparents.

Before Elliott left we administered two short pulses of radiation to the mass. Within forty-eight hours the veins of his neck had flattened, and his headache disappeared. It would buy enough time for him to make it to the West Coast and begin definitive treatment.

I contacted Jim Fox, reviewing Elliott's case in detail, and then sent him by overnight mail the pathology slides, copies of X-rays and operative report. The lymphoma, as I had feared, had spread to the bone marrow, but mercifully it had spared his liver and brain.

Elliott began the chemotherapy regimen four days after leaving Boston. He developed the expected side effects from the treatment: nausea, vomiting, hair loss, mouth blisters, diarrhea, and then less common complications. First was chemical pancreatitis, an inflammation of the pancreas from the drug L-asparaginase. He suffered weeks of severe abdominal pain that bored into his midback, and wild fluctuations in his blood sugar as insulin production fell. The high doses of chemotherapeutic drugs also injured the small vessels of his circulation. Fluid transited from his capillaries and swelled the soft tissues of his arms, legs, and face. This was eventually brought under control by aggressive administration of diuretics and restriction of his fluid intake.

The repeated courses of steroids resulted in painful necrosis of the bone of his right hip. It was decided that Elliott ultimately would need surgery and an artificial joint. The steroids also made his lungs a breeding ground for a fungus called aspergillus. This fungal infestation triggered spasms of his airways and severe air hunger. He needed oxygen, antibiotics, and bronchodilators.

Elliott stoically absorbed each awful side effect, and looked to his humor to diffuse his pain and fear. "I'm the Pillsbury Doughboy," he said when his body ballooned from the edema. "They say mature women like Susan love bald men," he quipped when his distinctive auburn hair was completely gone. With a raging fever and harsh cough from the fungal infection, his mouth ulcerated and his intestines unable to hold the little he took in, Elliott hoarsely concluded: "I think I finally outdid Job."

I stayed in close contact with Jim Fox by phone, fax, and e-mail. After receiving the clinical update, I would speak with Elliott. Our conversation developed a regular pattern, first mulling over the medical issues and then discussing his emotional state and the state of his family. I also visited him, using my frequent trips to scientific meetings in California as opportunities to see him in San Francisco or Sacramento.

Beyond clinical assistance, Elliott looked to me for hope. I told him all these complications were reversible, and we were very much on track with the lymphoma regimen. He began to ascribe to such words of support and reassurance a deeper significance, as if I were privy to a world of certainty beyond that of our senses. Susan, the hard-driving political operative, surprised me by also taking up this line. She regularly ended our joint discussions of his condition with the assertion: "If Jerry says it will be okay, then it will be okay, Elliott."

I felt deeply uncomfortable in such a role. I knew all too well how desperate we become facing life-threatening illness and its toxic treatments, and understood how we grasp at straws, wanting to believe that the doctor, with credentials and experience, can see the future clearly.

I tried to defuse their statements while still being encouraging, to gently restate the truth as I knew it, in scientific terms. I reiterated that the sum of the clinical data so far indicated that Elliott's chances were increasingly good that he would survive, but there were still major hurdles to overcome.

After his third course of the five-drug chemotherapy regimen the mass of lymph nodes disappeared in his chest. After the fifth course, no lymphoma cells were seen on his repeat bone-marrow biopsy.

With each positive advance, Susan and Elliott reaffirmed that I, like an oracle, had predicted everything would turn out fine, and my words were being proven true.

Elliott completed his eighteen months of intensive therapy. He then underwent complete restaging, with CAT scans of his chest and abdomen, bilateral bone marrow biopsies, and a spinal tap. There was no evidence of lymphoma. After so many invasive examinations, Elliott offered: "I always tested well, and this one was open book."

Elliott was declared to be in complete remission. It would take five years of follow-up before it was safe to state he was cured, because after that time, relapse was very rare.

"I will live with that uncertainty," Elliott asserted. "If I've learned anything from developing this disease, it is the fundamental uncertainty of all of life."

Two years later, in early June 1994, Elliott and his family visited Cambridge for his twenty-fifth Harvard reunion. I had never met his daughter, Tikva, now three years old. A petite and shy girl, she greeted me with a hesitant smile. Born after the fifth cycle of Elliott's therapy, when the lymphoma disappeared from his bone marrow, she was given her name as an expression of thanks. In Hebrew, *tikva* means "hope."

Elliott walked briskly with his family and me through Harvard Yard. Despite his artificial hip, he only occasionally depended on his cane to negotiate the inclines in our path. He was wearing sharply cut clothes he had purchased at Banana Republic in Berkeley to celebrate his complete remission: a white collarless shirt, beige linen pants, and a matching vest. His hair was thick and long, tied artfully in a ponytail. Susan remarked with a loving grin he was "Samson with his strength back."

Susan took Tikva and Benjamin for an early lunch while Elliott and I rested on the steps of Widener Library. We watched the preparations for commencement to be held the next day in the Yard, the stage arranged before Memorial Church where the president, deans, and tenured faculty would be seated facing the graduates.

Elliott was in a reflective mood, moved by his return to a place he cherished, where every student was told he was one of the chosen, graced to attend America's most prestigious university.

He candidly shared his recent thoughts with me. He allowed that for the first few months after returning to Israel he was thankful just to be alive, taking each day as a gift. To eat without mouth ulcers and diarrhea, to breath without oxygen pumped from a mask, to move his limbs without intravenous lines restraining them, this was enough to greet each morning with joy.

But now that he had fully resumed his former routine, writing at the *Israel Bulletin* and teaching film to undergraduates at the university, he was feeling deeply unsettled. During this reunion, he was realizing more forcefully than ever what had eluded him since leaving his alma mater. He wanted, finally, real success. Returned now to health, he was determined to obtain it.

I was aware we were moving into charged territory. We all want to succeed, and we usually define it in comparison to others, a problematic exercise. I feared that I might sound condescending or patronizing by saying this. Not knowing quite what to say, I remained silent.

"What have I accomplished?" Elliott continued as he gazed at the workmen hanging the rich crimson banners of each of Harvard's schools—law, medicine, business, divinity— from the poles of the stage. "This is what I have: a bimonthly column in a struggling Jewish magazine; two TV movies and countless unmade scripts; a part-time teaching job in cinema at Hebrew University.

"I know I almost died. It's not that I'm ungrateful for life. It's that I can't live on the edge every day, just thanking God and my doctors for my life. No one can live that way—it's a state of paralysis, a suspension of life. I have to deal with living again, in all its petty details—getting the kids to school and the car fixed and the taxes paid and the laundry done. And I have to deal with my larger issue—my desire to do something truly major.

"It was good to come back to Harvard, now, at this juncture in my life, after facing death. It energizes me to do what was always expected of me. And what I expected for myself."

He was thinking about finally writing a book. It was envisioned as a major work about the transformation of American culture. It would draw on the experiences he had had in a series of portraits of places in time: Brooklyn in the 1950s, when the American dream was like a collective unconscious; Harvard in the 1960s, the relinquishing of WASP propriety, of New England gentlemanliness, as authority was being challenged by the upheaval of Vietnam protests and experimentation with drugs; then the New York scene in the 1970s, the rebirth of careerism, the social climbing, the attempt to find an anchor and direction; L.A., meaning Hollywood, the wannabes, the groveling, the raw crassness of money and fame. And finally the West Coast in the 1990s, with the ascendancy of the wonks, computer nerds, and their venture people, who changed the way knowledge is received and processed by society.

"The experience of my cancer hasn't only made me want to do what I've always aimed to do—produce something substantial and important, a book that will be respected by the people whom I respect. I think I may have broken down the block to doing it. My illness has given me insights into myself that weren't apparent before."

Susan returned from lunch with Tikva and Benjamin, and we continued our stroll with them through the campus. We moved on to other subjects, the political situation, how the peace process was slowly but surely moving forward after the historic meeting between Rabin and Arafat. It was a time of hope and opportunity in Israel, and Elliott commented that, despite prior frustrations and failures, it was never too late for new beginnings.

One year after his Harvard reunion, Elliott had another opportunity to visit Boston. In addition to writing his biweekly column, he was now engaged in frequent travel as a public speaker. He had developed a reputation as a fresh voice in the Jewish intellectual scene. His commentaries drew on his considerable knowledge of Jewish history and tradition but added a modern secular slant. His subjects ranged from politics to cinema to books to religion. His readership in the *Israel Bulletin,* although select, was widely distributed throughout the Jewish world. He had addressed communities in Australia, Canada, and England already this year, and was now invited to New York to address a large rabbinical gathering. It was a special challenge, Elliott remarked, to "sermonize to the pros." He would come up to Boston midweek after his speech. Almost as an aside, he asked me to recheck his blood counts. On a routine visit last week with Dr. Levy, his general practitioner, his white blood cell count was noted to be just below normal.

"I'm at the tail end of a cold that I picked up from Tikva. Jeremy Levy thought this might have slightly depressed the number. You think it has anything to do with the lymphoma?"

I said I didn't. I agreed with Dr. Levy. Respiratory viruses often caused a minor diminution in the leukocyte count.

Elliott arrived looking strong and energized. There was a bronze color to his face from the Middle Eastern sun. His chest and shoulders were broad from his new passion, swimming. He no longer limped, having adapted to the artificial hip. We embraced forcefully, feeling the triumph that marked his survival. Pam and the kids welcomed him, as usual, with warm kisses.

Elliott did justice to a hearty homemade dinner, and rose early to read the *New York Times*. We spoke of the continuing move toward peace, how the redeployment in the West Bank was proceeding, and the chances that Rabin's Labor Party would triumph in next year's elections.

When we arrived at my office, my longtime assistant, Youngsun, greeted Elliott with great excitement, and spent much time inspecting his photographs of Benjamin and Tikva.

Two hours later I sat with Ned Waterman, the same pathologist who had reviewed the biopsy of Elliott's lymphoma. We systematically scanned the slide made from a single drop of Elliott's blood, which held thousands of white cells. Swimming among the normal white cells were several large, ragged forms. These unkempt cells had bloated nuclei and bright pink splinters littering their cytoplasm. I looked at the face of my colleague across the microscope, how his brow arched and the muscles of his cheeks tightened. The diagnosis could be made by a first-year medical student, the morphology of the large distorted cells was so distinctive. Elliott had acute leukemia.

I closed my eyes, the residual image of the leukemic cells lingering on my retinas. Then all I saw was deep blackness. I felt hollow, as if the darkness before my eyes had coursed down into the core of my being and emptied me of feeling. There was no anger, no pain, just a cold numbness, like the unfeeling shock of a person swiftly cut by a sharp knife who has no sensation of the wound.

Despite my emotional void, I immediately understood on a rational plane what had happened.

"Treatment-related leukemia" was the term applied to Elliott's condition, the cruel outcome of modern chemotherapy, which provided a life-saving result at first only to trigger, years later, a second, potentially fatal, disease in an unlucky few. The drugs that were given to Elliott to destroy the lymphoma had damaged the DNA of his normal bone marrow cells.

Most of these cells had died from the trauma, unable to survive with an impaired genetic program; a few had accumulated, by chance, the necessary mutations to lead to the opposite of cell death—the unrestricted growth of cancer.

I returned to my office, where Elliott was waiting for me. We had planned to go to lunch at Rebecca's Café, a gourmet fast-food place near the medical school. He had spent the morning at the Harvard Coop buying T-shirts for his kids and wandering around his beloved campus.

"It's incredible how fast they grow," Elliott remarked as I entered the office. "Last year at the reunion we bought them all sorts of Harvard outfits, and they've outgrown everything."

I agreed, saying kids grew like happy weeds, and then sat down. I looked into his soft blue eyes, knowing what they would soon see.

"Ell, I just returned from reviewing the slide of your blood test."

I paused. The cold emptiness that I had felt was now quickly replaced by searing pain.

I was tempted to hide behind euphemisms, to say there were some abnormalities noted and that further tests would be needed. I had thought that might ease him in to the news, the awful crushing news, that after all he had endured he now faced more, much more—a treatment as intensive and battering as any that existed in clinical medicine. To definitively eradicate the leukemia and cure him, chemotherapy would not be enough. He now required a bone marrow transplant.

But I knew, as before when I had informed him of his T-cell lymphoma, that it was best for him to know everything, as soon as possible, in honest detail.

"Elliott, it appears your white count is low because you've developed leukemia."

Elliott paused after my words and then nodded knowingly, as if he recognized a familiar face. I had expected him to flinch from the harsh blow just delivered, to break down in tears. I was fighting to prevent myself from doing so. But he sat still and silent.

I took his silence as assent to inform him of what was needed to cure him—a bone marrow transplant—and what that meant, since it was often misunderstood by laypeople. All the blood cells in his body would have to be destroyed. This would be accomplished by administering radiation, the kind of radiation that was called "total body" because it penetrated every millimeter of tissue, like the radiation from a nuclear bomb.

Once all his blood cells were destroyed, he would be given the most primitive marrow cells of a compatible donor. These primitive cells were called stem cells, because they grew into all the mature blood components—white cells, red cells, platelets—and could reconstitute his entire hematological system.

I waited for questions, but his silence continued, and I wondered if Elliott was really processing the information, whether it was all too much and he was overwhelmed.

"Am I clear, Ell? I know it's a lot, coming fast and furious."

He finally spoke.

"What if there is no match for me, no one compatible to provide the needed stem cells?"

It was clear that he did understand, all too well, because this was the key issue. Even if he passed through the treatment for the leukemia and entered remission, he could be left in a netherworld of waiting, unable to proceed to the transplant. Desperate options were then considered.

"If, God forbid, there is no match, from your family or the worldwide registry of marrow donors, then there are two options. One is conservative—to live in remission from your leukemia, knowing it will come back in months to years. You are healthy and functioning during that time, and, we hope, research advances give us a second curative path before the leukemia returns. The second option is fraught with risk—an unmatched transplant. With an unmatched transplant the stem cells grow into blood cells that will recognize the tissues of your body as foreign, and attack. This is 'graft-versus-host-disease'—the unmatched transplanted blood cells are the 'graft,' and they charge against your liver and skin and bowel, as the 'host.'"

"And the outcome of the battle?"

"Not usually in favor of the host."

I retreated from this discussion to focus on the most immediate step, treating his acute leukemia. I said we should operate under the assumption that he would have a compatible donor—Michael or Simon, his brothers, whose genetically related cells would be unlikely to cause a severe graft-versus-host reaction. I reviewed the logistics and latest statistics on matched transplants—at each point emphasizing the positive edge he might have: his general robust health, his relatively young age, the diagnosis of the leukemia early in its evolution. I was functioning as I usually functioned, as a clinician, with calm and expertise and honest optimism in the face of a complex and frightening disease. I thought I was transmitting to Elliott a sense of determination and authentic hope.

But Elliott seemed to move all the clinical science to the side, and surprised me with his response.

"What is your *choosh,* your sense, Jerry? Am I going to live?"

Choosh is a biblical Hebrew word, meaning "sense" or "feeling." It is onomatopoetic, capturing the sound of a rush of breath that emanates from the deep reaches of the spirit. It is a word that speaks not of rational deliberation and assessment, but of inner vision.

I paused, not expecting to have a *choosh* but an *opinion* as a sober clinician, one drawn from weighing the factors that went in his favor and those that did not.

But within me I had *felt,* not calculated, a reply.

"My *choosh* is good. I believe you will make it, that you're going to live."

I stood from my chair and hugged him tightly, tears now streaming down both our cheeks.

I wondered if I had gone mad, whether the anticipated pain and loss from imagining his death was so great that, after I rebounded from the numbing shock of the news, my rationality had collapsed and I was retreating into delusion. Who was I to pretend to be a prophet, to have extrasensory perception? What did my *choosh* mean in clinical reality? Was I indulging myself and my closest friend in a convenient lie?

But it was not a lie. I had felt it, clearly and strongly. Deep inside me was a prevailing calm. I clearly realized all the obstacles and uncertainties that lay ahead—the induction chemotherapy for the acute leukemia, the identification of a compatible match, the preparation with total body radiation for the transplant, the tense waiting to see if the graft of stem cells would take in his marrow space and grow to repopulate his blood, then the risk of graft-versus-host disease. All the while Elliott would be in a tenuous state—without an immune system—vulnerable to overwhelming and often deadly infections. He would be placed in an isolation room with special purified air and food, rare visitors allowed for short times and only under mask and gloves and gown, secluded as completely as possible from our ambient world of microbes while he lived without any bodily defenses.

But all these clinical realities faded under the powerful feeling that he would survive. I did not see light or hear words or otherwise hallucinate. And when I first heard his question, I assumed I would evade addressing it because in medical science *choosh* was meaningless.

But I had sensed that he would live, and it would have been a lie not to tell him.

"Let's call Susan now," I said, anxious to move away from the moment of mystical feeling and focus on logistics. "We should figure out the next steps with her."

"She's probably back from work by now," Elliott replied, looking at his watch.

I dialed their number in Jerusalem by heart, and as I listened to the flat ringing of the phone, wondered again if my experience of Elliott's illness was teaching me my limits.

Elliott decided to return to Jim Fox at Alta Bates Summit in Berkeley for the leukemia therapy and the marrow transplant. Its clinical unit was state-of-the-art; there was added comfort in knowing the nurses and the hospital routine; and the nearby resources of Susan's parents would again be of great help. Moreover, Jim had become not just his physician but his friend.

Susan flew to join Elliott in California, leaving Benjamin and Tikva in Jerusalem with Elliott's mother. The kids were in the middle of the school year, and it would be disruptive to take them out of class. They were informed that Daddy had to go into the hospital again. They reacted appropriately, disappointed but with understanding, since Daddy had spent so much time in and out of hospitals during their young lives.

Elliott received high doses of ara-C, a chemotherapy drug very effective against treatment-related leukemia but with terrible neurological side effects. He vomited for days despite powerful supportive anti-nausea medications, and then went into a swirl of vertigo as the ara-C temporarily shocked his cerebellum, the balance center of the brain. He could hardly speak, lying with his eyes closed and his head immobile. These side effects slowly passed over the course of two weeks. Then his hair fell out, his mouth blistered, his bowels ulcerated, and his blood counts fell. He developed streptococcal pneumonia and required oxygen and high doses of antibiotics. It was all too familiar.

Through each blow Susan clung to my words like a sure lifeline, repeating as a mantra: "Jerry's *choosh* is that Elliott is going to live."

After six weeks Elliott passed the first critical hurdle—the leukemia went into remission. He was discharged from the hospital. A week later, I was called by Elliott and Susan from her parents' apartment in San Francisco. Susan was the one to break the great news: Elliott's older brother, Michael, was an excellent match to be the marrow donor. She exuded determination like a tank commander leading a charge.

"On to the radiation. Then the transplant. Michael's cells are perfect! Just a few more steps forward. Everything will turn out fine, just as you predicted Jerry. Right, Elliott?"

Elliott had not spoken yet. There was a long pause before he affirmed Susan's words. Then, in a flat voice, he simply said: "Right. Everything will be fine."

Later that night the phone rang. I was in the kitchen, unloading the dinner dishes from the washer. It was well past ten, the kids asleep in bed, Pam reading in the den before we would retire for the night.

"Jerry, it's Elliott." His voice was hushed.

"You okay? Why are you whispering?"

"I don't want Susan to hear me. She's watching TV in the other room."

He paused and drew a deep breath. "I can't continue. I can't go ahead with the transplant."

I could hear him trying to control the quavering of his voice.

"Why not? You've done great so far. You've come through the leukemia treatment beautifully. Michael is a perfect match. We're almost there."

"I'm not sure why. . . ." he began to sob, "I just know . . . I can't . . . I can't."

He paused to collect himself, and then continued, his voice still shaking.

"Susan and you and my parents and Michael and Jim Fox—everyone just expects me to do it. But I can't . . . I can't fulfill your expectations."

I felt the distance of thousands of miles, the difficulty of finding the right words to reply without the benefit of seeing his face, touching his hand, following his eyes.

"Jerry, the transplant has become in my mind like writing my great novel or my major film script. The expectations that surround me—that have surrounded me all my life—everyone believing I could accomplish great things—it's all now focused on this. I just can't do it."

I paused to collect my thoughts. It was not my place to explore the degree of success or lack thereof in Elliott's life. That was not the critical issue now. What was critical was having him move ahead with the transplant, his only chance to be cured. I first tried an analytical approach, explaining to Elliott what I thought was happening to him psychologically, hoping the insight would comfort him and bolster his courage.

"Ell, it's normal to be frightened. Especially on the second go. It's like a soldier sent back to the front after surviving a first bombardment. You're still shell-shocked. You lose your nerve. That's natural, normal. I've seen this countless times with other people—a flood of self-doubt, all the secret insecurities rising to the surface and threatening to drown you.

"But you won't drown. We're all there supporting you, not with expectations but with love. I know Susan can be tough and drives you forward. It's her way of coping, her way of trying to keep herself, as well as you, intact."

"You don't understand, Jerry."

I heard him sigh a desperate, frustrated sigh.

"All my life I was expected to hit home runs, to slug it out of the park. Harvard. Yale. *Time.* Hollywood. But I'm not a home-run hitter. I hit singles—short grounders in the infield and pop flies. This time my life depends on a home run, and there isn't another chance at bat."

I continued to reassure him, saying that he was battle-fatigued, that Susan and I and Jim Fox and his parents were only trying to reinforce his will and confidence, not pressure him with expectations. But my words seemed hollow, and I feared would be ineffective.

I paused to regroup my thoughts, and could hear Elliott begin to sob again.

I tried to see the impending transplant from Elliott's perspective and then modify that perception to make it more manageable.

"My words are just words, Ell. I've only seen it from the other side of the bed, the doctor's side. But I don't think it has to be a home run to score. It can be a series of base hits, one single after another. It may sound like a silly metaphor, but think of it that way. Break it down into a series of manageable pieces, instead of seeing it as a daunting whole. You've already proven with the lymphoma and the leukemia that you have the strength to swing the bat. You don't have to prove anything more to yourself, to Susan or to—"

"Tell me your *choosh* about the transplant, Jerry," Elliott interrupted, his voice now more even and calm.

I sat silently, calling on my deepest feelings, seeking my inner sense of harmony or disharmony. It was again strange, because I did not resist his request. On a conscious level I wondered again whether this was all a game, my lack of resistance a way to extricate myself from a situation that had no ready solution. It was like a child's belief in the truth of fairy tales and the power of magic. I thought of the stories I had heard from my Hasidic relatives while growing up, of wonder rabbis, seers, diviners to whom the secret workings of time and space were revealed through angelic visitations and the study of mystical texts, kabbalah. I had been instructed by my parents to discount such tales as primitive and nonsensical. Was I assuming such a role for Elliott, or for me, or both?

But deep inside I had *felt* an answer and offered what I sensed, not what I knew.

"I feel you're going to make it, Elliott. I really do."

· · ·

Elliott returned to Jerusalem after the required one hundred days under observation in Berkeley. The marrow transplant had followed a remarkably smooth and uncomplicated course. His brother Michael's stem cells had found their niches in Elliott's emptied marrow space, and over six weeks began to spawn all the cells of Elliott's blood system. The growth factor G-CSF was given to expedite the maturation of the transplanted white cells, which reached normal numbers by week ten. There was no sign of graft-versus-host disease, and the medications that were used to prevent this complication were soon to be tapered off.

We had spoken several times each week during these critical one hundred days. After assessing the progress of the transplant, we discussed the biology and medical science that gave rise to the procedure. Elliott had brought a laptop computer into his isolation room, and in addition to e-mail and writing, had researched the history of the technique on the Web.

The Nobel Prize in Physiology or Medicine was awarded in 1990 to E. Donnall Thomas of the University of Washington at Seattle for developing marrow transplantation. It was the culmination of a remarkable story. The first eleven patients treated by Dr. Thomas had died within a few weeks. It was an extraordinary act of determination to persevere, to believe that the barriers to transplantation of human bone marrow could be surmounted.

The biology of the process is similarly remarkable. The rare stem cells, present only at a frequency of 1 in 10,000 donated marrow cells, could be infused into a recipient's vein, circulate through the body, home specifically to the emptied marrow space, and then grow to fully reconstitute our entire blood system—its billions and billions of cells that comprise our immune defenses, oxygen-carrying capacity, and clotting functions. It is a testimony to Nature's astounding regenerative powers.

Elliott commented that beyond the exceptional history and biology was another dramatic dimension to marrow transplantation, one likely experienced only by the fortunate recipient. It was expressed by a verse from Leviticus: "The life of the flesh is in the blood." Within him, flowing in every tissue space—heart and brain and muscle and gut—were the life-giving blood cells of his brother Michael.

"I feel as if I've been reborn, like I participated in a new form of Creation, joining the hand of God with the hand of Man."

While I rejoiced in Elliott's metaphor, I somberly remembered what it had taken to bring bone marrow transplantation to the sophisticated state it now enjoyed. Some two decades earlier, when I was a hematology fellow at UCLA, bone marrow transplant was still in its infancy. Dr. Thomas had just passed the first hurdles and achieved sustained grafts. A transplant unit was established in our department. There were many, many failures that now would have been successes. Little was known about how to optimally administer total body irradiation and the adjunctive support to carry a patient through the procedure. There were no available growth factors like G-CSF to stimulate white blood cell production from stem cells and accelerate the return of the body's defenses. As a fellow on the transplant ward, I watched impotently as patient after patient developed overwhelming infections and died. The medication Elliott was taking, cyclosporine, to modulate the "education" of the grafted cells, so they gradually "learned" to tolerate their new home and not rebel in a tantrum of graft-versus-host disease, this too did not exist when I was in training. The ravages of this awful graft-versus-host reaction, with liver damage, diarrhea, and skin sloughing, were all too frequent then. If a patient survived, he was generally left incapacitated.

Elliott, my beloved friend, husband of Susan, father of Benjamin and Tikva, had been given back his life because of the stubborn commitment to research of physicians like Donnall Thomas. Science did change the world, fundamentally and for the better.

Elliott called me from Jerusalem three weeks after his return to tell me that Susan and his parents were planning a "survival party." Pam and I were invited, although they doubted we could come.

I told him we would celebrate in spirit from Boston, and toast the miracle of science that had returned him to family and friends.

"You saw it all along, Jerry. Your *choosh* was that I would make it."

I felt uncomfortable. I wanted to celebrate the triumph of medical research, not vague mystical intuitions.

"I don't know what my *choosh* meant, Ell. I did feel it, but perhaps it was just a delusion, a psychological mechanism to help me cope with the nightmare you were in."

Elliott paused and then replied thoughtfully.

"I've come to believe more in that mystical dimension, Jerry. Isolated all those days, my own cells forever gone, the stem cells of Michael growing into my new blood, I had a strange *choosh* of my own.

"I sensed it wasn't only coincidence that Anne Albright brought us together, but that she envisioned you as my brother, and then my two 'brothers'—you in spirit and Michael in flesh—saved my life. I felt a visceral connection to you, to Anne, to all the people who have loved and cared for me during my life. I felt this at the moment of the transplant. I felt as if all your spirits were being infused into me along with the marrow. As much as Michael's stem cells revitalized my body, your spirits breathed life again into my soul."

We left it at that, making these mystical experiences a part of the history between us, and moved on to talk about work-related things.

"I haven't figured out what I want to do yet," Elliott confided. "Whether it makes sense to continue at the *Bulletin* and on the lecture circuit, or do something different.

"I'm trying to understand what 'success' means in my life. That's not easy. It's a struggle. I've been thinking about how I measure success in light of what I've been through.

"When I couldn't hold a pen to write, focus my eyes to see, or even lift my head to speak, I realized that performing such simple acts then would have been a 'great' success. It's a cliché but true that you don't appreciate what you have until it's gone.

"I learned in yeshiva years ago the question posed by the Talmud: *Mi adam ashir?* Who is the wealthy man? And the rabbi's response: '*Hoo sameach im ha-chelko.*' He who rejoices in his portion.

"I rarely deeply rejoiced in my portion before. But in my isolation room, as my new blood was being created, I was able to write my column again. And I *rejoiced* in doing it.

"You know my first article was about my leukemia and the transplant. After it appeared in the *Bulletin,* I was deluged with mail. So many readers wrote, not only wishing me a speedy recovery and sending words of support, but affirming how powerfully my ideas affected them. I realized that sometimes they do cheer you when you get on first base, that singles do count in the game.

"I have hardly lost my ambition. I still want to write a book of substance, of significance. But I see the reason for my ambition differently this second time. Above all, I have to find it satisfying, I should rejoice in it. I want to look inward, not outside myself, for a measure of its success."

I understood Elliott's struggle. The desire for greatness, to be recognized for your achievements, was an insatiable worm that gnawed at your consciousness, invaded your dreams. Who didn't suffer its effects? Driven to do more, make more, rise higher. But it was a fruitless climb because there was no real summit.

I knew this from my perch as a physician, witnessing the moment when the seemingly endless climb is abruptly, unexpectedly, irreversibly halted by the advent of life's end. As death looms, so much of the success that we have lusted for appears useless and vain.

There are, of course, lasting achievements in life. I thought of the success of Donnall Thomas. He was certainly driven by ambition, pushed forward by the desire to conquer Nature's barriers and do what had not before been possible. And he had been awarded the Nobel Prize, science's highest honor. But that worldly acclaim paled before a greater honor— the legacy that he had created for Elliott and others like him who now could live.

"It's very hard to live by one's own inner standards, Ell."

"Probably impossible. But I'll try. And when I feel myself slipping back, I'll tell myself to reflect on how I felt during the transplant, how my life was so brutally constrained, how my days were literally numbered."

"Literally numbered?" I wasn't sure what Elliott meant.

"Yes. Each day on rounds Jim and the nurses would number the days: day zero was the day my blood was destroyed by the total body irradiation. Then day one was the infusion of Michael's stem cells. Each subsequent day was numbered. It was a weird experience, to listen to Jim Fox count at my bedside and declare to the medical team: 'Today is day fourteen post-transplant, vital signs stable, no sign yet of recovery of the graft.'

"I was both terrified and hopeful—terrified because I knew Jim could be counting the last days of my life, but hopeful because it felt like he might be numbering the days of my second creation. And if I survived, I knew I would be reborn in a unique way, not like the infant with a blank slate, but with memory and insight from all that I experienced."

Elliott's words brought to my mind the verses from Psalm 90, a psalm of life and death. It is recited in the synagogue to begin the mournful service of *yizkor*, the service of remembrance of those loved ones who are gone. I saw myself then, standing deep in prayer, my eyes closed, seeking insight from memory. This time the words spoke to me not of loss but of gain:

> *The stream of human life is like a dream;*
> *In the morning, it is as grass, sprouting, fresh;*
> *In the morning, it blossoms and flourishes;*
> *but by evening, it is cut down and withers. . . .*
> *Our years come to an end like a fleeting whisper.*
> *The days of our years may total seventy;*
> *if we are exceptionally strong, perhaps eighty;*
> *but all their pride and glory is toil and falsehood,*
> *and, severed quickly, we fly away. . . .*
> *So teach us to number our days that we may attain a heart of wisdom.*

caring across borders:
aging parents in another country

JULIA ALVAREZ

Abruptly, in the winter of 2002, my elderly parents announced to their four daughters that they were returning "home" to the Dominican Republic. This was almost as much of a shock as their announcement when we were little girls that we were leaving the island for New York City. Back then, my father had gotten involved in an underground plot against the dictatorship that had been discovered, and we were forced to leave the country in a hurry. But that emigration had not been by choice and we had left all together.

Now, forty-two years later, Mami and Papi were choosing to go back without us. Just at the time in their lives, seventy-five and eighty-six, when they would most need our care as their health became more fragile, they were choosing to put distance between us. At the time in their daughters' lives, I should add, when we had our hands full with careers finally off the ground and busy family lives. Caring for them in a nearby city would have been challenge enough. Caring for them in a whole other country without the infrastructure to help us would be tough.

In an odd way, this was poetic justice—or injustice, as the daughters saw it. The tables were now being turned on us! As young women, my sisters and I had wanted to be free of their old-world control. We had insisted on moving away to attend college and to work at jobs in distant cities. We had fought with them to have apartments, friends, bodies, lives of our own.

And yet, no matter how far we wandered, we always came back to one another. "The only ones who will always be there for you will be your familia," Mami warned every time we struck out on our own. Her prediction had proven to have some truth. Anybody got sick, we were all there. Anybody had a problem, the phones began ringing. An eleventh-hour caravan hit the road to rescue whomever was in trouble. Although the four daughters had become American women with professions, husbands, children, minds of our own—in that one aspect of our lives we remained unadulterated Dominicanas: nuestra familia was sacrosanct.

"But we can't go with you," we argued with them, about their imminent move. Our jobs, our husbands, our children were here.

"What if you get sick or lonesome?" We peppered them with questions and warned against certain consequences.

But they were firm. They wanted to return to what they had known in their childhood and young adult lives, to a slower, warmer, Spanish speaking world without the pressure of a life in English in a big city.

But it would be a life without *us*! The Gretel question in all their daughters' hearts was, *Why did you bring us here if you were going to abandon us later on?* "We'll be American orphans," we commiserated by phone. But how could we argue with what amounted to a deathbed wish? This was how they wanted to live out the last few years of their lives.

You'd think we were little kids, not grown women in our fifties. But inevitably like all progeny around parents, we turned into their children, thinking about their choices as they related to us. Actually, though we talked in terms of ourselves, it was a larger loss we were feeling. If, as my mother swore, she and Papi were never coming back to the States, how would they participate in the ongoing family story: the lives of their grandchildren, American kids who barely spoke Spanish, who felt out of place in the Dominican Republic? Not only were we losing our parents in our American lives, but our children were losing their grandparents.

We gathered together in their apartment in New York City the weekend before their departure. On Sunday, a cold and gray March day, the time came for my husband and I to drive back to Vermont. My mother, always one to avoid pain with activity, stayed upstairs in their apartment packing. But my father rode down in the elevator with us to stand on the sidewalk and wave as we drove away.

I climbed into the car, willing myself not to cry and make it harder on all of us. Never again would I see my papi standing before that apartment building, a dear, familiar face in a city of strangers. In his gray fedora hat and black overcoat, he already looked outdated, a throwback to another century. The hole in my heart was so big, I thought I'd fall through it. Of course, I was also grieving a future loss: the final leave-taking that would make permanent orphans of the four of us.

As we pulled away, I rolled down the window. The tradition back on the island was for children to ask for their parents' blessing when they parted.

But when we arrived in this country, this ritual along with others had fallen by the wayside. No way we wanted our parents giving us blessings before our spiffy new friends at boarding school or camp or later in college. But now, there was nothing I wanted more than to feel the balm of my father's blessing on my head.

"La bendición, Papi!" I hollered. Folks on the street turned to see what the commotion was about—a scene I would have avoided at all costs as a young teen.

From the curb, my father lifted his hand. I saw the condensation of his breath in the air more than I heard his reply.

Soon after they settled in Santiago, our warnings—wise, parental children that we had become under their tutelage—proved true. My mother banged her leg against a piece of furniture, and a screw that had been inserted in her ankle years back worked itself loose and to the surface; the suppurating wound would not heal. There were long-distance phone calls, Mami crying that she feared her leg would have to be amputated, complaints about long waiting lines in clinics. The doctor who finally saw her told her that she would need surgery: the screw had to come out.

Meanwhile, Papi's memory had begun to fade noticeably. Certain behaviors that had seemed odd in New York City—an obsession with the tiniest slights, paranoid fantasies that my mother was having an affair, that something lost had been stolen—became even more exaggerated. There were consultation calls with doctors. The diagnosis we suspected was confirmed: my father was sinking into Alzheimer's.

My sisters and I were thrown for a loop. How were we going to manage? My husband, an ophthalmologist, tried to convince Mami to come to Vermont and have the loose screw removed by a colleague at our local hospital where he also operates. She and Papi could stay with us until they could travel back again. We would take care of Papi. We would take care of her.

"No, no, no!" She burst into tears. She was fearful of being trapped here, too ill to travel back, too feeble to be self-reliant, having to die in a country full of strangers.

"We have to honor their wishes," was the litany we heard stereophonically and emphatically from all of my sisters who called within hours of my mother hanging up. The family gossip mill was alive and well—no loose screw there. It turned out that Mami had called them, tearfully relating that my husband and I were trying to force her to come to Vermont.

"Brace yourself," my husband warned. "This is just chapter one." After eighteen years living with a writer, he knew how to pick his metaphors. After eighteen years as a member of our family, he knew how the plot was likely to go.

But even without my sisters' outraged chorus, I would have honored Mami's wishes. Short of her actually endangering herself and Papi, what else could I do? Elderly parents might be as fragile as infants, as unreasoning as toddlers, as unable to manage their affairs as children, but they are still our parents. And in our old Latino culture that term carries even more weight—our viejitos command our total respeto by virtue of their age and experience. There is a popular saying in the Dominican Republic: The devil knows more because he is old than because he is the devil.

But the problem remained: How were my sisters and I going to care for our ailing viejitos? Any one of us could take a week or two off, but what my parents needed was ongoing, hands-on care. Unlike in the States, there is no senior care system available in the Dominican Republic, or rather, the system in place is the extended familia. But after forty-two years away, my parents had not established those critical bonds with that new generation of familia who could help them out. In addition, they had moved back to their childhood hometown of Santiago, in the interior, far away from the capital where our maternal cousins who did feel a connection to Mami and Papi were located.

So began the tough challenge that continues to this day of how to care for our aging parents. Many of the problems our American friends face with their elderly parents (Is it safe for them to live unsupervised at home? Can they manage their medications on their own? What happens if there is an emergency?), my sisters and I are also facing, compounded by the fact that Mami and Papi are far away in a developing country where even the basic services—electricity, telephone, water—are iffy. Our parents have fallen between the cracks of two worlds: no longer can they subscribe to that old-world familial care system nor can they partake of senior care in this First World, choices which might include home-care services or an assisted-living facility or even a small condo close enough to one of their four daughters so that she can stop by, and then call up the other three to relate what happened today to Mami and Papi.

During that first crisis in which Mami needed surgery and Papi was anxious when he couldn't find her in the house because he'd forgotten the explanation that she was in the hospital, we, the sisters, fell into some old patterns. First of all, though I painted the other three with the broad brush of consensus—all agreeing that my husband and I should not abduct my parents to Vermont—there were variations in their vehemence. All our familial life, we had differed, often squabbled (and made up)—four strong-willed, divergent opinions, dancing around the principals, Mami and Papi. Why would this stage be any different? Years back, a hospice worker once told me how families expect a different kind of behavior from an ill or dying member. Some sudden turnabout. A wish or need that never got fulfilled by that person suddenly granted. The tidy resolution that we've come to expect from our only other experience of narrative: novels and movies. But that's not what happens, she explained. "People die the way they live: messily and in character."

This also applies to family dynamics around aging or ailing relations. Since childhood each of the daughters has had our specific role in the

family. The eldest has always been the family negotiator who pulls everyone together with her therapy skills. I, the second oldest, am the writer
in the family who goes off on her own to create. Then, the third sister
is the nurturing, self-sacrificing giver of the family. Finally, the baby gets
to be spoiled and fussed over. Years ago, when the four sisters discovered
Little Women, we were astonished, especially since my mother claimed she
had never read the novel. Not just our birth order but our personalities
and even the first letters of our names (Meg, Maury; Joe, Julia; Elizabeth,
Estela; Amy, Ana) matched those of the March sisters.

Not surprisingly, during that first crisis, the Alvarez sisters fell into our
accustomed roles. The oldest called up wanting to talk about what was going on, how we felt about it, what we should do. Before we knew it, the
third sister was already winging her way down to the island. The youngest,
a single mother, could not leave her daughter alone to go down and be
with our parents. In fact, my mother scolded her for even thinking about
traveling. She had her hands full already. She would get sick if she didn't
take care of herself. Meanwhile, I was setting out on a book tour, feeling
guilty that I was carrying on with my professional commitments while
dropping the ball on the personal front.

In part, my husband had urged me not to hover and hyperventilate.
He had spoken with Mami's physician in Santiago. The procedure would
be quite minor. Mami would be kept in the hospital overnight just so she
could get extra care. "You sisters get so worked up!" my husband said,
shaking his head. "What are you going to do when a real big thing happens?"

But although I could let him talk reason to my head, my heart felt
divided. Care in our dramatic, emotive family as well as our culture also
includes *showing* you care. Every night from hotel rooms, I'd call down to
Santiago, where my oldest sister had joined the third sister. After getting
the up-to-date news—Mami's procedure had gone well, Papi's medication
had been increased to manage his anxiety over my mother's absence—I'd
call the baby sister, who like me was feeling torn that she had not gone
down to join the others.

This is what comes of Mami and Papi making this choice, we complained to each other, only because we didn't want to blame ourselves

anymore. But there was truth to our feelings—as there usually is to the feelings that well up when there is an illness in the family. Suppressing them or judging them just adds to the tension and trouble. But of course, tact and timing are of the essence. Everyone is ill at ease when someone is ill in a family. Everyone needs caring if not medical care.

I confess that yes, along with worry and sadness and missing them, I also felt a slight resentfulness: they had made a choice which required that we give up our lives here to go take care of them there. My husband and I had the opposite experience with his parents. In their later years, they had moved close by to make it easier for us, still engaged in an active work life, to take care of them. Having them five minutes away meant we could drop by almost daily, share several meals a week, be a phone call away in an emergency, attend to their needs on an ongoing basis. Their choice seemed considerate, an understanding of the natural cycle and their place in it.

But my parents, my dear viejitos, were operating according to an old-world order which was their formative culture. They needed to go back to their homeland, their mother tongue, their culture as they approached death and a literal return to the earth. "As flowers depart / To see their mother-root when they have blown," George Herbert describes it in a poem. Back home, the extended family unit is the rule. In fact, the choice my in-laws had made—to hook themselves onto our nuclear family—would have already been in place back where my parents came from. The old people live next door if not in the same house with their children and grandchildren. They are invested in the same family business from which they all draw their income, and which the old people have turned over to their sons, rarely to their daughters—why my feminist sisters and I would find it difficult to return to that Dominican family structure.

But it's more than that. My sisters and I were formed in a different world where mobility scatters us all, and self-reliance is not just a virtue but a way to survive. We have to make our own living, take care of ourselves in this country. But as first-generation immigrants, we are also creatures of that old world, its costumbres, valores, and tradiciones. An old world that now holds two of our dearest beings on this planet—another reason that it would be impossible to let go of that world. Not that complete assimilation in our new country has ever been a choice for any one of us.

At every stage of our lives, my sisters and I have had to figure out how to integrate these two worlds. As we take on the role of caretakers and elders, we will each have to find the balance that works for us. The old culture holds up the abnegating, self-sacrificing woman who gives up everything to take care of her parents, her husband, her children. The new culture is more Cordelia-like in its approach, prudent in its promises, avoiding the expansive gesture that plays beautifully in the early scenes, but often fizzles out when the crisis comes. I admire the expansiveness and generosity of the former; the straightforwardness and accountability of the latter.

In fact, that Shakespeare play, *King Lear*, has come to mean more and more to me as my family enters this caretaking stage of our lives. The old can be as demanding and peevish as children, and as with children, we must set limits in order to curb the understandable self-centeredness of those who are needy, often sick, lonely, and powerless. By the same token, compassion flows out to them. Do we haggle over how much they need? "O, reason not the need," King Lear cries out to one of his daughters who promised him everything but now quibbles over each thing he asks for. Though I've tried to be clear with myself about what I can reasonably give my parents, when I hear their frail voices on the other end of the phone, the heart floods with feeling, and I yearn to give myself over to them.

As for our roles in the family, part of growing up and growing older involves expanding beyond those limiting paradigms that hobbled us when we were younger. Why we moved to those distant cities, struck out on our own in order to become more fully ourselves. Away from my sisters, I've discovered that I can be the nurturer, the good listener with therapeutic advice, as well as the one who needs babying and spoiling. Part of the challenge of taking care of my increasingly absent father and fragile, childlike mother is not to let the old roles dictate our choices. Or to alienate us into stances. If for no other reason than we, sisters, need each other's help more than ever.

But sometimes we find ourselves chafing against our old assignments.

Childhood rivalries crop up, and we're back to square one, four "little women" in full-blown regression.

It seems the baby sister (all of fifty-one years old) calls our mother nightly before she goes to bed. A sort of tucking each other in. The conversations always begin the same way. My sister asks, "How is my little mother?" And my mother responds, "How is my little girl?"

A few days ago, I happened to call up one night and my mother answered, "Is this my little girl?"

"Yes, this is one of your little girls," I said, more sharply than I intended. Jealousy over parental favoritism does not end when you stop needing favors from them.

In fact, it's my mother who more and more is the little girl with four mamas, each one trying to figure out how to be the best caretaker she can be. How to work in concert when the balance that is right for one sister might not work for another? No one can make that judgment for me, not even my husband, whose reasoned German Lutheran approach I've tried to emulate, only to end up dissolving into my own messy Caribbean self. What seems an unbearable sacrifice or too great a demand to one might be another's wish or desire or need. I recall how the third sister recently told my husband that she would be going down every few weeks to check in on my parents. My husband responded that there was no need to be a sacrificial lamb.

"That's insulting!" my sister told him. "It's my privilege to go down."

Where do I stand? Somewhere between these two—I won't call them extremes but poles of how to take care of our viejitos.

Sometimes I am more Cordelia. Sometimes a chip off the old Latina familia.

A few weeks before this past Thanksgiving, I called my parents to wish them happy anniversary, which falls earlier in the month. Although it was only afternoon, I woke my mother up. This was very unlike my mother to be taking a nap in the middle of the day. "Well, I didn't have anything to do," she explained tearfully. "Your father just wants to lie in bed sleeping. He didn't even wish me a happy anniversary."

My heart was in my throat. "Mami, remember: he doesn't remember."

That was no excuse. "It's our fifty-ninth anniversary." Her voice grew faint; she must have turned. No doubt, Papi was lying on the other side of the bed. She wanted him to hear her.

"What are your plans for Thanksgiving?" I asked, wanting to get her thoughts on to another holiday. Through the gossip mill, I'd heard that one of my sisters (you guessed it, number three) would be going down to be with them.

"No, she's not coming until the week after," my mother explained. "It's a bad time to travel. Besides the kids'll be there."

"So, you'll be all alone?"

"That's okay," she said, perking up. "Your father and I don't like turkey. Right, Papi, we don't like turkey?"

He must have stirred awake. "What?" As usual, he couldn't retain what he heard or figure out what to say. "Put him on," I asked my mother. I wanted to wish him a happy anniversary as well. But my father insisted it wasn't his anniversary. "Yes, it is, Papi. Plus, I want you to repeat after me so that Mami can hear you, okay? Happy anniversary, Mami. Say it, Papi, 'HAPPY ANNIVERSARY, MAMI.'"

"Happy anniversary, Mami," he repeated.

I could hear the pleasure in her voice. "Ay, Pitou." Her pet name for him. "Happy anniversary to you, too."

When I hung up, I called my husband at work. I couldn't stand the thought of my viejitos all alone for Thanksgiving, even if they didn't like turkey. I was going to go online to try to find a last-minute ticket. Did he want to come along?

"What do you mean?" he snapped. "I haven't seen them since June either. I miss them, too!"

It's not just the Alvarezes who have touchy tempers.

Of course, when we arrived in Santiago on Thursday, Mami was bright and breezy. Papi seemed more alert than the last sister to have seen them (number one) had reported. In fact, both parents were doing reasonably well. "I told you so," my husband told me. But still, he was glad to be spending Thanksgiving with them. His own parents had died within five months of each other five years earlier. "You and Papi are the only parents I have now," he told my mother that night, making Mami and me both burst into tears.

. . .

Returning back to Vermont from Santiago on Monday, we had our usual long layover between flights. I always use the time to call the sisters with the latest news of how our parents are doing. I'm also under longstanding orders, which began back when we were teenagers, to call Mami to tell her we got in safely. I have to laugh because what is my eighty-year-old ailing mami, who refuses to travel to the States, going to do if I call her from Atlanta to say my plane had to make a crash landing? Besides, by the time we are actually home in our house in Vermont, it's way past midnight and I am not about to wake her up in the middle of the night to tell her I'm home. So, I usually call her from Newark or JFK and pretend we're already back in Vermont.

"That was quick," she exclaimed at the other end.

"Yes," I agreed, hoping some blaring airport announcement wouldn't come on. "And tomorrow another visitor," I reminded her. Sister number three was headed down the Tuesday after Thanksgiving.

"I see more of you here than I ever did in New York," my mother remarked, which was the truth. Because of the long distances and the cost of travel, each of us now spends one to two weeks with them several times a year instead of those quick weekend trips shared with other relatives.

"It's like I got all my little girls back by moving here." She giggled. The thought crossed my mind: Had our canny mami done this on purpose?

"You're going to get sick of us," I teased her.

"Never. The only ones who will always be here for me are my daughters." Her voice had grown weepy. A new twist on an old warning. This, too, I would tell the others.

In parting, I asked for the blessing that had now become our routine. "La bendición, Mami."

"La bendición," she repeated. This had been happening lately. She'd forget how it went. Instead of blessing me, she was asking me to bless her.

What's the difference, I thought, and gave her my blessing. But then, always the daughter, I reminded her: "Now it's your turn, Mami. Bless me back."

called them vitamins

STEPHEN YADZINSKI

When I was twelve, growing up in Buffalo, New York, my dad and I would get in the car on sunny Sunday afternoons and drive the quarter mile or so to our local middle school. The school was always quiet, and the sky was a crisp, clear blue. Around the back of the building, near the rear of the parking lot, the school's high brick walls had no windows. Dad had found the place years before, and knew it was the world's best spot to hit a tennis ball against the wall.

I remember watching my dad, amazed at his ability to volley with himself and almost never miss. For the half hour or so he played, I would listen to the sounds of the game: the racket hitting the ball, the ball hitting the wall, the rustle of dried fall leaves blowing in a corner, my dad breathing hard. In the middle of the wall was a metal No Parking sign, and to keep the game interesting, Dad would aim for it. When he hit the sign, a loud *clack* would echo through the lot.

The image of Dad playing his solitary game, looking back on it now, seems odd. If you came upon the scene you might suspect my dad's feet were somehow glued to the pavement, or that maybe it was part of the game for him to not move his feet at all. He moved like a strange machine, metronomically swinging his arms from his hips, hitting the ball from one side of himself to the other. Of course, occasionally, he did miss the ball. When that happened, and the fuzzy green ball bounced past him, he was no more able to retrieve it than if he'd hit the ball on the roof. The truth is, if he tried to move his feet very much at all, he would have fallen flat on his face.

Years earlier, during a routine physical exam, doctors observed what they called my dad's "unusually slow reflex reactions." At the time, no one—not the doctors, not my mother, not even Dad himself—thought much of the observation. It was nothing more than a passing comment during a quick exam.

My father and mother were at the top of their fields then as professional musicians in the Buffalo Philharmonic Orchestra. The Philharmonic was then one of the most respected orchestras in the country, and my parents each won their jobs at young ages. They had been recently married and expecting their first child, my older brother, Gregory. Life was, they thought, good.

I was born four years later, and by that time my parents' marriage was in serious trouble. They had begun to disagree frequently, especially about money. When I was two years old, Dad took a yearlong sabbatical from the Philharmonic and taught music theory in San Diego. Shortly after he returned, Mom filed for divorce. Dad moved to a small apartment nearby, and Greg and I lived with our mom for the next eight years. When the Philharmonic started having financial difficulties, Mom found a better paying job with the Atlanta Symphony Orchestra. Greg and I moved to Georgia with her, and Dad moved back to our family home.

The daughter of a violinmaker, my mother began playing the violin when she was just three years old, and she never once considered another career. Dad says Mom was always the best musician onstage. A unique performer, she rarely practiced and almost never remembered the music she played. Seven days after her retirement, ending a forty-five-year career, I asked Mom what the program was the night of her last performance. She could not remember. Mom considered her playing a job; her passion for the music had left her long before.

My father is different: he loves everything about music. During his prime, he was among the best clarinet players in the country. The night after I was born, Dad played Carnegie Hall, and the music director, Michael Tilson Thomas, announced my birth to the orchestra. In his midtwenties, my father toured Europe with the avant-garde composer Lukas Foss, performing Foss's experimental *Echoi*. Throughout his career, Dad played with people as well known as Leonard Bernstein, Pablo Casals, Henri Mancini, and even once with the Grateful Dead. By any standard, my dad had a fantastic career and an even more incredible talent. To this day, music is always around him.

After two years in Atlanta, my brother and I were miserable. Even though I made friends, had birthday parties, and played Little League Baseball, I always felt like an outsider. I began suffering from chronic headaches and had nightmares. Greg, wanting more than anything to be with his friends in Buffalo, became depressed. Our classmates called us "Yankees." Before moving to Atlanta, my brother and I had never thought about the cultural differences between North and South, and we were surprised to find so many popular references to the Civil War. I remember seeing a large bumper sticker that had a cartoon drawing of a Rebel soldier yelling, "Forget, Hell No!" Stone Mountain Park, a major attraction just sixteen miles outside Atlanta, presented a laser light show over a giant carving of Robert E. Lee and other Confederate leaders sculpted into the side of a massive granite hill. Once, driving home along a country road from swimming at Lake Lanier, I caught a glimpse of Klansmen gathered in a field, erecting a large, wooden, fabric-wrapped cross.

Greg and I came to the same conclusion: there was no point to our living in Atlanta, no reason for making it work. The rift was between our parents, we figured, and neither of us understood why our lives should be so disrupted. After all, our father still lived in our childhood home, my best friend still lived across the street, and Greg's best friend still lived just two blocks away. Greg, who was considered the mature and reasonable one, lobbied Mom and Dad for our return to Buffalo. It was not a matter of who we wanted to live with, he explained to our parents, but rather, *where* we wanted to live.

After months of discussion, our parents gave us a choice: Atlanta or Buffalo, Mom or Dad. Mom asked my brother and me separately. I sat on a stool in our small kitchen. "More than anything," she said, "I want you and your brother to be happy. If you want, you can move back to Buffalo." I knew my brother had already decided to go, and I didn't hesitate: I chose Buffalo. My mom began to sob. Crying, my voice just beginning to change and crack, I yelled, "What did you expect me to say?" She didn't answer. My mom knew how hard living in Buffalo would be. She knew something I was only beginning to comprehend: My dad was sick, and he wasn't going to get better.

That September I started sixth grade in Buffalo, my brother started high school nearby, and Dad started walking with a cane. Still, for a while, life in Buffalo was more or less normal. By the end of that first year, though, Dad's strength and ability to balance were significantly degraded. Walking became especially difficult, and soon my father began to fall. It was frightening, especially when it happened in public: at the grocery store, or in a restaurant, even once onstage before a concert. He always fell the same way. The cane would slip, his legs would buckle, and down he'd go. Hitting the ground so hard must have hurt, but he never let on. My brother and I stood him up, brushed him off, and gathered the contents of his ever present soft-sided briefcase. Strewn about the floor were pens, keys, pills, and change. We did our best to ignore everyone's stares. Once, he fell so hard he broke some ribs.

Doctors were perplexed by Dad's illness. His first symptom was numbness in his feet and legs, and some specialists believed my father was afflicted with a rare, as yet undocumented form of multiple sclerosis. This was impossible to confirm, and Dad continued to search for other possible diagnoses. After several years, a dozen or so doctors, and countless tests, he finally found his answer. While working with a clinic in New York City that specialized in neurological medicine for musicians, an MRI revealed damage to Dad's spinal cord. The results were highly unusual—the location of the injury was consistent with a dramatic accident or fall, but there was no such event to which Dad could point. The clinic referred Dad to Dr. Fielding, a Manhattan neurosurgeon who was among the best spinal cord experts in the world. After reviewing the results of the MRI and performing a quick physical exam, Dr. Fielding said, "That's the weirdest goddamned thing I've ever seen. I don't know how you did it, but I can't fix it." Then he added, "Don't you let anyone tell you it's MS, because it's not. Now put your clothes back on, I have patients waiting."

My dad asked the doctor to show him where the damage was. "Can you point to it, on my neck, with your fingers?" Dr. Fielding rapped the back of my dad's neck with his knuckle and said, "Right there, right between C-5 and C-6. You tell them to look there again, they'll find it." Sure enough, high on his neck and deep inside, my dad's spinal cord was catastrophically damaged. There was no apparent cause or cure.

No one's personality is suited to the transformation from health to sickness, but my dad's was a particularly bad match. A lifelong workaholic, Dad kept unusual hours. He slept during the day and played for the Philharmonic or taught university students in the evenings. Through the night, he composed music and sometimes listened to opera, *loud.* He'd take phone calls at all hours from musician friends who knew he'd be up. Sometimes he made home improvements, whatever small job he could manage in his declining health, unclogging a sink or changing an electrical outlet. Once, I woke to the sound of a circular saw cutting wood and came downstairs. I told him to quit it. It was a school night.

We ate out most nights, usually at a Greek restaurant a couple miles from our house. Dad's cane was almost useless by then, and getting into the restaurant with him was a real challenge. Everyone around him knew he needed a wheelchair, but Dad was not ready to acknowledge this. So I would hold out my arm for Dad, locking my elbow in a right angle. He would grab my forearm and lean on me. We would then move slowly together, a half step at a time, until we reached our table. The chore was embarrassing for me, but not hard.

When I was fifteen, my brother went off to college, and my dad and I were left alone in our house together. Small chores—writing, holding utensils, and tying his shoes—were more and more difficult for Dad, and I began helping him get ready for work. Before each performance, I buttoned his shirt, clipped his tie, and tied his shoes. I remember standing in his dimly lit bedroom, working quickly on the small tuxedo buttons. Pinching and fastening his collar's last button, I felt the warm skin of his neck. I felt uncomfortable, as if some subtle violation were being committed. As I worked under his chin, he looked away, avoiding my eyes. Standing awkwardly and not quite steady, he once said, "My hands feel like I'm wearing gloves."

Oversized prescription bottles filled with big, pink, oblong-shaped pills came into the house. I unscrewed the childproofed tops for him and dumped their contents into the front pocket of Dad's nylon briefcase. He called his pain medication "vitamins."

"Son," he would say, "I need a vitamin, would you mind reaching down in my bag and grabbing one for me?" Invariably, the pill I chose had dust and fuzz stuck to it. He'd blow it off and swallow the pill.

When I remember my dad playing the clarinet, the word fragile comes to mind—not soaring, or technical, or strong—but *fragile*. His hands were quitting him, and no one knew exactly why. Soon he'd no longer be able to play. This was difficult for me to comprehend. His instruments and music had always seemed so *permanent* to me. When I was four, Dad and I played a duet of "Frère Jacques" on his clarinets. The bass clarinet's black wood, silver keys, and small upturned bell were striking and rich—luscious even. Dad took pictures that day. Wearing plaid pants and a white turtleneck, I stood on my tiptoes and was then almost as tall as the instrument. In the photos, I am laughing.

Dad invented a key for his bass clarinet that made playing easier for a while, but as his illness progressed, the slight advantage the key provided stopped working. A memory of notes he couldn't play was just around the corner, and Dad had invested too much time—and love—into his music to suffer such an indignity. He later told me it was better to retire five years too early than five minutes too late.

It irritated my father to watch sports luminaries, past their prime, eke just one more season out, only to diminish their reputation. Dad saw himself in those players and believed his reality was cruel, but he also knew there was nothing anyone could do about it. And so, at the age of forty-eight, twenty-five years into his professional career, my dad retired from the Buffalo Philharmonic. That day, Dad arrived home at the same time he always did, early afternoon, shortly after I got home from school. With him were his two saxophones, four clarinets, and the bass clarinet. It was rare for all the instruments to be in the house at the same time. Usually he kept a couple clarinets and a saxophone or two in his locker backstage at Kleinhans Music Hall, the philharmonic's home in Buffalo. Quietly, Dad placed the seven instruments in the back of a large walk-in closet outside his bedroom. I never heard him play again. A year later, Dad sold his instruments. We needed the money. Besides, he said, if no one played them, the clarinets would crack.

Dad got his first scooter shortly before his retirement. A small, three-wheeled machine with a large black vinyl seat, its front wheel rotated beneath a yellow plastic cover, inspiring us to call it the Canary. The scooter itself was heavy and awkward, but it made moving around the house easier for Dad. He continued teaching part-time at the University of Buffalo and drove to campus most days. In the evenings, he'd pull our Subaru wagon into the driveway and turn off its engine. Dad would sit in the car for a long time; he called it "re-charging his battery." After a while, he would honk the horn.

I'd emerge from my bedroom, run downstairs, and grab the fifty-five-pound Canary from the back of the silver wagon. I would carry the scooter inside our house and leave it perched atop the four steps in our back hallway. Returning to my room, I would hear the bash of our old wooden door as it swung open, crashing into the wall. The plaster behind the door handle was cracked and broken, and the door's glass window would rattle in its frame. My dad never intended to be loud or careless, he simply couldn't help it. Dad would grab the small stairway's metal railing tightly with his right hand, and then with his left hand, take hold of his left pant leg. Pulling, he would drag his limp and unresponsive left foot over the step's metal-trimmed edge. He would slide his right hand up the railing and then use his left hand again to haul his right foot up to the same step. Three more steps, and three more times he would repeat these motions. The entire event took ten minutes. At the top, Dad would sit quietly in the seat of his Canary, once again recharging his battery.

By the time I turned seventeen, Dad could no longer climb the back hallway steps by himself. I would crouch down by his side, and he would lean on me. I'd grab his ankles and lift his feet, first one and then the next. We'd move together, one half step at a time. At the top, I'd help him turn and land in his scooter. It was not for another year, until *after* I had left for college, that Dad allowed my brother and me to build the ramp he so obviously needed.

In my senior year of high school, Dad relied on me more and more. I did his laundry, cut his meat, opened cans of soup, and poured his Tab into the big plastic tumblers he could drink from without spilling. I got the mail, bought his newspapers, and went grocery shopping. Occasionally, I helped my dad shower. No one cooked. We ate Le Menu frozen dinners or went out.

Housework became almost impossible for Dad to do. I suggested re-organizing the kitchen so he could unload the dishwasher and get his own glasses. He became angry and didn't want to talk about it. I was angry, too. Mundane conversations—especially his simple requests for help, like getting the mail or fetching a pen from across the room—turned increasingly confrontational. Often, alone in my room upstairs, I'd hear his voice call out, "Stephen!" The sound penetrated every room of the house. He always needed something.

Sometimes, sitting in school or at a friend's house, I'd think I heard Dad's voice calling faintly, in the distance. My right shoulder began twitching constantly. I was anxious and had trouble sleeping. Every night, I'd fall asleep with my black-and-white TV tuned to reruns of the *Benny Hill Show*. I'd wake to "The Star-Spangled Banner" playing quietly as the station went off the air, and watch the desaturated American flag billow over slow-motion images of Niagara Falls.

I spent as much time away from home as possible. I played guitar in a rock band, had a girlfriend, and spent hours working alone in the basement darkroom I built. I developed landscape pictures, and thought about living out West someday. On the weekends, friends and I drove to the edge of Buffalo and bought alcohol from a convenience store, known among teenagers for its liberal identification policies. We'd bring the cases of beer back to my house and sneak them upstairs when Dad was in the bathroom or on the phone. It wasn't hard. We'd throw small parties and hang out the windows smoking cigarettes and marijuana. So long as we kept quiet, listening to music or watching a movie, there was no chance of getting caught. Dad couldn't walk upstairs. Most teenagers like to get one over on their parents, and I was no different. Our parties helped me to feel independent, normal, like any regular kid.

One night that year, I woke to my dad's voice: "Stephen," he cried, "Could you come down here please? I need some help, son."

Cursing him under my breath, I got out of bed. I knew he had fallen.

I was mad, but I hurried. Downstairs, standing in my underwear and half asleep, I saw my dad lying on the kitchen floor. He had lost his balance reaching for a cup of tea. There was a puddle by the stove. It was quiet. Only the light over the sink was on. My dad's scooter was between us.

"I'm fine," he said. "I just need a hand." He rolled from his side onto his back, and looked at me apologetically. I looked away.

"Don't move," I said. I grabbed him under the arms, probably too hard. I jerked his body off the floor and dropped him into the seat of his scooter. A moment later I was upstairs. I didn't wipe up the tea or bother to ask if he was okay. I didn't say a word. I was finished sharing his illness.

A few years ago, my wife, Susanna, and I visited Dad in Buffalo. He still lives in the same old house. To help cover the mortgage, Dad rents out the second floor bedrooms to graduate students studying performance at the University. Almost all the renters study the clarinet.

In the fourteen years since I left for college, much has changed around the house: there's a new automatic door and a professionally built ramp; Dad's specially equipped van is parked in the driveway; and Dad has a helper dog, a sheltie named Pegasus. She gets the mail, can fetch the remote from under a chair, and can bring Dad a pair of shoes from across the room. Dad jokes that she's an improvement over a seventeen-year-old kid: she doesn't talk back.

During that trip, Susanna and I took Dad to an appointment with his neurologist. At the medical center, Dad moved quickly in his scooter through the long, curving halls. The red wall-to-wall carpet muffled the noise of the chair's electric motor, and the tungsten bulbs lining the ceiling cast a dim orange light throughout the windowless space.

Dad pulled up to his doctor's office and waited for Susanna and me to catch up. He couldn't open the door. It opened the wrong way, toward him, and it was too heavy anyway. I got the door and Dad drove into the brightly lit office. He set off for the receptionist's window, accidentally knocking into a chair along the way. The window's sliding glass door was positioned high on the wall, and Dad's forehead was just barely even with its sill. Leaning out the window, a woman handed several forms attached to a clipboard down to my dad. He drove to where Susanna and I were sitting. I was busy reading an article in the *Smithsonian* about an artist who made miniature versions of ancient bridges. Dad handed me the forms and a pen, and dictated his answers to me. A few minutes later, a nurse called his name.

Susanna and I sat together in the waiting room, talking quietly. She asked about Dad, and what it was like living with him back then, when I was a kid. Did I take him to the doctor frequently? Is he worse today than he was before? Things I don't tend to discuss. I answered as best I could.

As we talked, the heavy office door opened. A man in his midfifties sitting in a powered wheelchair drove into the waiting room. A boy of about twelve followed quickly behind. Like my dad, the man drove straight to the receptionist's window and got some forms, then headed to where his son was sitting. I watched them closely. The man's hands worked well. He held a pen, filled out the forms, and then flipped casually through a magazine while he waited. The boy was quiet, had an intelligent face, and looked relaxed and comfortable in the waiting room.

The man's wheelchair was well maintained and nearly spotless. A yellow backpack hung off the back of his chair. I imagined it was full of the things he might need throughout the day: a fresh pair of socks, a warm hat, maybe a pair of gloves.

When I was in high school, we didn't make plans. There were no family meetings, no discussions about Dad's illness. We didn't know what would happen if Dad fell so hard he was seriously hurt, or if he got so sick he needed more help than we could give. We were all just winging it.

I could blame Dad for not allowing my mother, my brother, and me to help him in more substantial ways than we did. We could have talked to his doctors more, helped him come to terms with his degenerating condition. We could have pushed him to anticipate the progression of his disease and make plans for the future. Dad has told me that one of his greatest regrets is not having built a ramp into the house while I still lived with him—we should have forced him to do this. The truth is, though, none of us wanted to be more involved than we already were. We saw ourselves as short-timers, doing what was necessary until we could each slip away—Mom into divorce, and my brother and I into adulthood.

Since I left for college, I've come home only for short, three-day visits. Friends of the family have been critical of me for not helping Dad more. I understand. Looking at my father today, slumped over his scooter, straining to keep his head upright, you'd think he needs me. But the truth is, he never wanted my help. He simply wanted to live his life, to play his clarinets, to walk from the driveway to the house without needing someone to lift his feet for him. For a while, I was there to help him get through. I was a tool, like his scooter. And then I was finished. Anyone would have done what I did.

ruth

JUSTINE PICARDIE

Recently, I've spent a bit of time in hospital as a patient. Nothing life-threatening, but even so, it's left me feeling pretty low. I've been trying to untangle the reasons why, and I'm beginning to think that the main reason isn't the aftereffects of the anesthetic, or the discomfort of surgery, but something else entirely. What I want is to talk to my sister again; a want that feels as urgent as a child's. I long for her to hold my hand, and understand that I'm scared, in the way that only a sister can do, because you know each other through and through; but she's not here anymore, she's gone. . . .

Actually, that's not quite true. Ruth is right here—inside my head, inside my heart—but she died in 1997, of breast cancer, at the age of thirty-three. She had been diagnosed less than a year previously, and the disease spread swiftly, inexorably, to her bones, her lungs, her liver, her brain. Ruth had given birth to twins in August 1995, so her husband, Matt, had his arms full with two babies at the same time as trying to earn a living for all of them, which meant that I tended to be the one who accompanied my sister to hospital for consultations and treatment. It just seemed to work better that way.

I hesitate about using the word *carer* to describe my role in the eleven months between Ruth's diagnosis and death. It doesn't sound right somehow, but I suppose that's what I was (along with my mother, and several others who were dear to Ruth, trying to stop the unraveling of her life, as death came closer each day). I cared for my sister; sometimes I cared so much that it felt overwhelming, a tidal wave of love, and also of misery at

being unable to keep her from dying. And, at the same time, as if on au-
topilot, I did the practical stuff: chasing up doctors, arguing with hospital
bureaucrats, seeking second opinions from professors of oncology; though
in retrospect, all that was probably a form of self-preservation, as much a
way to stop myself from going mad as anything else.

I was at work the day she was diagnosed. She'd gone to that first hospital appointment alone—it had seemed like a routine one, to get a lump
in her breast looked at, one that she'd already been told by several doctors was benign. Anyway, she rang me in the magazine office where I was
working at the time, and said, "I've got breast cancer." Ruth was crying,
and I thought, *This is impossible, this can't be happening, not to my sister, not
to me,* but I said, instantly, "It's going to be okay, I promise, I'm not going
to let you die."

It wasn't okay, of course, and I could do nothing to stop the disease
that was spreading inside her, stealthily consuming her, immune to prayers
or pleas or medicine or miracles. All I could do was care for Ruth, whole-
heartedly; by which I mean, to be with her, and to love her and to tell
her that I loved her, and that life would never be the same without her.
Isn't that what caring really means, in the end? That, and trying to make
sure she had enough money, so that she didn't worry about bills; because
love doesn't pay the mortgage. . . . Oh, and bring bunches of lavender and
sweet peas for her, and fresh supplies of chocolate brownies or lemon cake;
those were important, too, because being with Ruth taught me that small
pleasures can be as precious at the end of a life as the big stuff. That's why
she asked me to go clothes shopping with her, or to a film, if she was feeling up to it, something that would make her laugh.

And when I think back to that terrible, unforgettable time, it did
include laughter, however black the circumstances. We laughed until we
wept on her first night in hospital, after Ruth's initial session of chemotherapy, when the nurses, in their wisdom, put her in a bed next to
a woman dying, alone, of breast cancer. (It wasn't the nearness of death
that made us laugh, hands stuffed into our mouths, tears rolling down our
faces, but the thought of attempting to obey the instructions of the medical staff, who reiterated to Ruth that, "The most important thing is to be

positive." And then the nurses closed the curtains around that nameless woman in the adjacent bed, who seemed to have no visitors, no one who cared enough to be with her in her last hours. I wish now that I hadn't been frightened of this woman's rasping breath, of the tubes and oxygen machine; that I had gone to her, if only for a moment, and held her hand in mine. This is one of many failures that I remember from the time, all of which I remain ashamed of.)

One of the strange things about Ruth's cancer was that she didn't seem ill, until she started having the chemotherapy, which made her very sick indeed. I'd sit with her while the drugs were administered intravenously, and it felt like I was watching my sister being poisoned. But she didn't really want to talk about any of that, at least not very often. (And anyway, my feelings about her treatment were not the point; it was her that was undergoing chemotherapy, not me, and I knew how draining it was for her to deal with other people's expressions of misery about her illness; it was almost as bad as the ones who used to behave as if nothing was wrong, or tell her not to worry, their aunt's friend had survived breast cancer.) So I used to read to her instead; mostly she asked for *Pippi Longstocking*, which was her favorite childhood book, the one that I'd read to her long ago, before she was old enough to read, when we were still children, and had shared a bedroom, me on the top bunk, her on the bottom.

It's a wonderful story by Astrid Lindgren, as you may already know, about a nine-year-old girl who lives alone without her parents; Pippi's father is a ship's captain who has disappeared at sea during a storm; her mother is dead, though no reason is given why. "Pippi's mother had died when Pippi was just a tiny baby lying in her cradle and howling so dreadfully that no one could come near," Lindgren writes. "Pippi believed that her mother now lived somewhere up in Heaven and looked down on her little girl through a hole in it. Pippi often used to wave up to her and say, 'Don't worry, I can look after myself!'"

Ruth had always had something of Pippi about her as a child, I'd thought: she was brave and bold and unconventional, and she'd worn her wild curly hair in two unruly braids for school. She was strong, too, like Pippi: she swam most days, and cycled to work, even when she was preg-

nant with the twins. As her older sister—her only sister—I knew all her
strengths, and admired them, but I knew what frightened her, too. I knew
that she hated the sight of blood, particularly her own, and that the endless needles and drips in the hospital were a torment to her. I knew, too,
that even though she sometimes gave the impression of being as fearless
as Pippi Longstocking ("Don't worry, I can look after myself!"), she was
frightened of dying, because she could not bear the thought of leaving her
children, as Pippi's mother had done before her. But she faced this savage
truth, because she had to; even though it sometimes made her howl as
dreadfully as the baby Pippi did, when no one could come near.

And sometimes, Ruth was angry, and I knew that I needed to let her
be angry; that soothing words were not what she needed then, for she had
much to anger her. (Perhaps it is easier to do this for your sister than your
husband or wife; or not easier, not exactly, but somehow, you can accept
that this is how it is; that when your sister is sick, you can be strong for her;
and you don't expect her to be stoic or good-tempered, not in the way
that you might expect from a partner, say, the parent of your children.)
The month before she died, when she was finally admitted to hospital,
having developed what the doctors politely termed "disinhibited behavior" (a symptom of the tumor in her brain), she raged against everyone
who tried to keep her there, including me, and finally discharged herself
and walked all the way back to her house, very fast, followed by me and
my mother and her husband; an anxious family retinue that simply fueled
her rage.

At home, at last, she opened her bedroom window to the summer's
day outside, and shouted, "I'm dead, I'm dead, I'm dead!" And then she
went to bed, exhausted, and stayed there, her white face turned to the wall.
I sat with her, and massaged lavender oil into her poor, wasted body, and
stroked her shorn head, the dark curls all gone now, along with so much
else. She talked very little, though I hoped we had already said everything
to one another, in the previous weeks, before the brain tumor had affected
her speech. I had told her that she would always be with me; she said she
knew that, though she worried that I would be lonely when she was gone,
because you could never replace a sister, not like a wife, and we cried, even

as we spoke about how death was not a final ending. But later, as she lay stilled and silent in her bed, while August turned into September, I felt that she was on a lonely journey where I could not accompany her, nor give her the help that she needed (as if in forewarning of the void that separates the living and the dead).

Finally, Ruth was admitted into a hospice, a strangely peaceful place, close to her home in south London. Her room was on the ground floor, with doors that opened onto a beautiful walled garden where late summer roses bloomed, and a heavily fruited mulberry tree dripped dark red juice, like blood, onto the ground. On sunny afternoons in the Indian summer, as the shadows were lengthening, we sat outside on a bench beside the mulberry tree, and she lay down, with her head in my lap. She was so tired, and I wanted to give her my strength, to give her everything, but there was nothing I could do but love her. It was simple, unconditional; unbearable, at times, but it had to be borne. I loved my sister; I love her still.

Ruth died in the night in the last week of September. She had been in terrible pain, it had suddenly risen up and taken hold of her; the pain was going to kill her, she said, and so I told the nurses to give her more morphine, to ease the awful suffering and agony. I sat beside her, then lay next to her for a while, my arms around her, and whispered into her ear. "I love you, I love you, I love you." I said the words to her, over and over again, like an incantation, and then she opened her eyes, and took the oxygen mask from her mouth, just for a few seconds, and said, "I love you, too."

Those were her last words to me. And then she died. My sister died, and none of my caring could prevent her going, and all her fierce love for her children was not enough to keep her alive. Because that's one of the things you learn about caring: it's huge, but it doesn't work miracles, despite being miraculously limitless.

Since then, I haven't stopped caring about my sister. I care that she's not here today, when I want her in the most childlike of ways. I care that she did not see her children last month, on their eleventh birthday; I care that she is not with them today, and every other day, day after day after day. I have grown older but not grown careless; I know that love is the most precious of things, that we should cherish those we love, in the knowledge that in the end, our care for them means everything, even when it seems to come to nothing; for caring, like love, entwines us around each other, threading through our lives, and into death, as well.

I cared for my sister. She cared for me. In the end, it all comes down to this.

notes on accepting care

ANDREW SOLOMON

I had a good run at being a caretaker in the years immediately before my first mental breakdown. My mother was dying of cancer, and in retrospect, I could have done better with the caretaking, because I was twenty-five and full of ambivalence about the role reversal. I wanted to be there for my mother, but I was young and had my own life to live, and was angry at fate for getting in the way of my happiness. Sometimes, that translated into anger at my mother, and so we argued. Sometimes the anger turned on my father, because he was so unconditional in the care he took of my mother. My father's lack of ambivalence seemed to throw my own mixed feelings into sharp relief, and he cared so much for my mother and so little for anything else that was happening that I felt trampled. I was too young to understand the urgency of impending loss. He would ask me to come home every time she went through the slightest difficulty, without much regard for the ways I thought such diligence was wrecking my life. My father had always been the great problem solver; anything we brought to him, he had always made better with love or money or intelligence or compassion, and my mother's illness was the one thing he failed to cure. I wanted him to handle it, and I was grief-stricken that he couldn't, and, childishly, I resented the powerlessness implicit in his asking me to help ameliorate what he could not fix.

Despite all that, I did a lot for my mother during her two-year battle with cancer. She was not only the person my father loved most, but also the person I loved most. I called her every day, often several times a day, and came home to New York every month or so from London, where I was living. I went to great lengths to get things for her that I thought she might like (English books, her favorite peonies), and kept the house merry with a cavalcade of carefully chosen gifts. I consulted with my father about her medical care—which was mostly a matter of affirming his beliefs, but it took time and thought to do it convincingly. I tried to fly the banner of good cheer when her moods sank. As her situation became more serious, my own ambivalence was mitigated, and the reality of the loss became incontrovertible. I mourned in a visible way that was difficult for everyone but that must have assuaged any concern she might have had about how deeply she was loved. I ultimately left England and moved back to New York to be near her during her final months.

It would be a gross lie to say that I didn't express my own sorrow while she was alive, sorrow about her impending demise and about the cavernous void that the very prospect of that loss opened within me, but I was holding onto sanity and didn't realize how tenuous my grasp was. After she died, the slippage accelerated into darkness and sadness and blunted despair. As I sank, I kept calling out to my father, who had taken such good care of my mother; but he was negotiating his own anguished landscape, and he was calling out to me, too, and neither of us could hear the other. We groped along in mutual pitilessness and self-pity, exhausted and alone. Flashes of romantic love pulled me out of this dire condition, but they were misguided at best, and often seemed like new locations to which I could tether my misery rather than like actual life experiences to which real and appropriate sentiments might attach.

I began developing symptoms of mental illness. I didn't understand what was happening, but I knew I could not face it alone. In desperation, and in the absence of my mother, I turned to my needy father with a need that trumped his own. He rose to the occasion, and our subsequent famous relationship has been built on that fact. I considered myself a caretaking person, but I had no idea what solicitude really entailed until I had been its object.

My father had been nurturing enough when I was little, but attending to the ill was my mother's department, as was exploring the complex and frightening world of emotions. She was the one who kept track of feelings, and who attempted gentle resolutions of life's upsets and frustrations. My father was jolly and cheerful and slightly vague about the details of our lives. He loved us beyond measure, but it was not his full-time job to do so. I didn't know what capacities he had until I watched him with my mother in those final years, and I didn't fully comprehend the power of such nurturance until I was its target. In retrospect, this seems strange. I don't know to what extent my father changed and to what extent he was simply manifesting what had always been his underlying character. Both things are true, but their proportion remains obscure to me, and, I would think, to him. What is clear is that when the time came, my wobbling self discovered a foundation of granite in my father's compassion.

I wrote a book, *The Noonday Demon: An Atlas of Depression,* that includes the specifics of my illness, and I will say here only that in retrospect, I hardly believe that I stayed alive through it. I couldn't feed myself for days at a time. My sleep was fitful and full of painful dreams, and when I was awake I wanted only to sleep again. I knew that my state was ludicrous, that I had an essentially good life and that all this despair was a folly, which only made me feel worse. I found it frightening to be alive; I was as anxious as if every second were a final exam, as sad as if everyone I loved were dying, as numb as if I were embedded in polar ice. If I had been able to think of a passive way to give up on life, I'd have done it in a flash; what stood between suicide and me was how much effort it would have taken effectively to annihilate myself. My inability to shower became a symbol of the laughable extent of my disability; I felt paralyzed by the time I had swung my legs over the side of the bed to sit up. The prospect of walking the requisite twenty steps, turning on the water, adjusting for temperature, getting under that beating water, using soap and shampoo, getting out, turning the water off, drying myself—it was almost inconceivable. All over the world, people were taking showers. Why could I not be one of them? Then I would reflect that those people also had families and jobs and bank accounts and passports and dinner plans and problems, even cancer and hunger and the death of children, and isolating loneliness and failure. By then, the idea of a shower would have come to seem foolish and unrealistic and I would be relieved to pull my feet back up into bed, so I could lie in safety and feel ridiculous.

Always at the back of my mind, a calm and clear voice said, don't be so maudlin; don't do anything melodramatic. Take off your clothes, put on your pajamas, go to bed; in the morning, get up, get dressed, and do whatever it is that you're supposed to do. I heard that voice all the time, that voice like my mother's. My father is not depressive and does not find life difficult unless he is compassing difficult situations. He has rough moments, and the years after my mother died were extremely painful and profoundly sad for him, but my father is always highly functional: functioning is his default condition. My mother functioned nearly as well as my father, but for her it was a constant battle that involved a great deal of pushing herself through. She didn't have the acute depressive symptoms I developed, but her vitality was an exercise of will. A trace of melancholy peeked out behind even her gladdest smiles, but she never indulged that side of herself. With a steely self-discipline, she kept all our lives running merrily on course, including her own; she was living proof that being sad didn't prevent you from being happy. It was my father who could take care of me, but it was the memory of my mother that told me how to take care of myself.

Like most people, I did not want help when I started feeling horrible. I wanted to get through it on my own. Indeed, I wanted to protect the privacy of my sorrow. It took months of deterioration before I finally caved and went to see a psychopharmacologist. My first day on medication, I moved into my father's apartment. My father was almost seventy, and most men of that age cannot easily tolerate complete shifts in their lives. His flexibility of mind and spirit allowed him to understand how he could be my mainstay through rough times, and his courage helped him to be that mainstay. He canceled all plans so he could stay in with me, night after night after night. He was relentlessly cheerful and never flagged (at least in front of me) in his conviction that I would soon be well, despite copious signs to the contrary. He led a cheering section, and also dealt with the pragmatics, cutting up my dinner for me when using a fork and knife was entirely beyond me. I would tell him not to feed me, that I wasn't five, at which he would recount how he felt when I was a child, and he would make me promise, jesting, to cut up his lamb chops when he was old and had lost his teeth; but despite that joke there was nothing reciprocal about the situation. We achieved a symbiosis in which he was perfectly tolerant, and I tried to be perfectly acquiescent. I found the situation somewhat humiliating, and he claimed that he couldn't see why.

Since my depression followed a diurnal rhythm, at its worst in the morning and at its best just before bedtime, I would rise to some of his good humor at night. Before bed, Xanaxed out but not yet asleep, I would joke with him about my sorry state, and that rare intimacy that surrounds illness would make itself felt in the room, and sometimes I would feel too much and begin to cry again, and then it was time to turn off the lights and go back to oblivion. Some evenings, my father read to me from the same books he had read when I was a child. I would stop him. "Not long ago, I was writing my novel," I said. "I used to work twelve hours and then go to four parties in an evening. What's happened?" My father would assure me, sunnily, that I would able to do it all again soon. He could as well have told me that I would be able to build myself a helicopter out of cookie dough and fly it to Neptune, so clear did it seem to me that the life I used to live was now definitively over.

During this first serious depression, I had to embark on a book tour for the aforementioned novel, *A Stone Boat,* which dealt in loosely keyed form with my mother's death. The publisher had scheduled me to go to the West Coast for a series of readings. I had started on medication, but was still in the first throes of treatment, that wonderful period when you get all the side effects but not yet any of the desirable results. I remember lying in bed in a state of unremitting panic because I knew I couldn't go, even though I had dreamed all my life of publishing a successful novel and couldn't forgo this opportunity. Squashed between my Scylla and Charybdis, I suddenly thought of asking my father for help, again. In the course of my entire life, I'd never known him to miss a day of work except once, when I was in second grade and he had fallen and cut his face so badly he had to go to the hospital; and then during the months when my mother was sick. I found my own illness both comical and deplorable and I hated the idea of disrupting his life anymore, but it felt like my only choice, and when I asked him to come with me, he assented instantly and gladly. I remember the wave of relief, the feeling that under his vigilant eye it would all be fine, that he would take care of me and that I was going to allow it. My breathing changed: even the prospect of travel did not send me back into panicked, shallow inhalations.

My father took me to California. He got me on and off the plane and to the hotel. So drugged-up that I was almost asleep, I could manage these changes, which would have been inconceivable a week earlier under any circumstances. I knew that the more I managed to do, the less I would want to die. During our first dinner in San Francisco, I suddenly felt my depression lift. I chose my own food. I had been spending days on end with my father, but I had no idea what had been happening in his life, besides me; depression is a disease of self-obsession. We talked that night as though we were catching up after months apart. The next morning, the misery returned in full force, but at least I had enjoyed a brief window of normality. My father came with me for the next week, and in the week after that, he called me every few hours. I was never alone for long. The knowledge that I was loved did not in itself constitute a cure, but without it I could not have completed the book tour. My father had made wellness seem like a plausible object for which I could rationally hold out hope. Without his tender care, I would have found a place to lie down in the woods until I froze and died. Recovery depends enormously on support. If there is a rational piece of you that survives the distortions of illness, that piece knows whether there is anything to get well for. The constant reminders of my father's love made me feel that if I could recuperate, a life of some value awaited me on the other side. I couldn't feel that value, but I knew that it was there, and that was a strong motivator for getting better.

Even so, I was angry at my father some of the time, angry in an irrational, miserable way. I was enraged at the world and at fate and at my own brain, and my father was a handy outlet for this anger. I told him he was pushing me too hard, or not hard enough. I was young, comparatively, and still aching from the loss of my mother, and from the end of a deep romantic relationship and the elusiveness of a new one. He meant his assurances to be uplifting, but sometimes they felt like trivializations of my very real condition. I was not going to be fine and I wanted him to acknowledge that. I was indebted to him, but my appreciation teetered constantly at the brink of ingratitude. Just as I was beginning to get better, he said something that upset me, and I heard my voice go shrill and my words grow sharp. I could see the trace of apologetic, perplexed recoil in my father. I breathed deeply, and said, "I'm sorry. I promised not to yell at you and not to be manipulative, and I'm sorry." In depression, when we need love more than ever, we are at our least lovable. Depressed people stick pins into their own life rafts. I exploited my depression as an opportunity to put up a wall around myself, through which I could sometimes receive but seldom express any positive emotion.

While receiving care is a great deal better than not receiving care, it's a lot worse than not needing care. My father's kindness at some level reminded me of my own helplessness. I was upset by the needs my depression created, even when those needs were being met unstintingly. In later depressive episodes, I understood what was going on a great deal better, and I depended less on a single source. By then, I had built up a better network. Friends eased the burden on my father, and eventually I found love and had a supportive partner to split the work. In depression, you make what the disinterested world judges unreasonable demands on the people around you, and friends and even lovers often don't have the stamina or knowledge or inclination to cope. If you're lucky, some people will surprise you with their adaptability. You communicate what you can and you hope. Slowly, I've learned to take people for who they are. Some can process depression or other illness right up front, and some can't, and I no longer blame the people who are allergic to clinical desolation. Most people are repelled by the unhappiness of others. Few can cope with the idea of a depression divorced from external circumstances; most would prefer to think that if you're suffering, it's with good reason and subject to logical resolution based on a direct address to that reason. There are things that only others with the same wounds can understand; I know from my unsympathetic pre-depressive days how incomprehensible depression is to those who haven't had it. Spouses, parents, children, and friends can be brought down themselves, and they do not want to be close to measureless pain. Depression is extremely contagious, and smart people try not to expose themselves to it any more than necessary—though experience can serve as a vaccine and native resilience an immunity. My father resisted catching my illness both because of his inborn buoyancy and because he needed his own good spirits to ensure mine.

No one can do anything but beg for help (if that) at the lowest depths of a major depression, but once help is provided, it must also be accepted. We would all like Prozac or intensive cognitive-behavioral therapy to do the trick, but in my experience, we have to help it along. One can't just pull himself up by his bootstraps when he can't even get out of bed to find his boots, but on the other hand one can't just shift the burden of recovery to medical interventions. A depressed person cannot be drawn out of his misery with love (though he can sometimes be distracted). Even if a caretaker cannot shine light on the darkness, he can, sometimes, manage to join someone in the woeful place where he resides, so he is not alone there. It is not pleasant to sit still in the darkness of another person's mind, though it is almost worse to watch the decay of that mind from outside.

So many people have wondered what to do for depressed friends and relatives; it's perhaps the question most frequently asked of me when I lecture, and the form in which it's presented is usually that a depressed friend or spouse or parent or child rejects help and claims to want to be alone. Don't believe such people for a second. What they mean is that they find it stressful and exhausting to fulfill any expectations, and that social interaction may be more than they can handle, and that they can't demonstrate an instant recovery response upon the proffering of affection, and that they feel guilty. Sometimes, depressed people cannot bear to have another person in the room with them because the presence of such a person feels like an implied demand. In that case, sit in the next room. But soothe their isolation. Do it with cups of tea or long talks or by staying nearby and silent, or in whatever way suits the circumstances. And do it willingly, without expectation of a quick return on the investment. You can't undepress another person, but don't leave. Someone who feels truly alone is bereft of hope, and that is the path to suicide and ultimate despair.

When frantic people ask how they might emerge from their own depressions, I think how much love would help. The unavailability of love to some of these people seems a worse disability than their illness itself. After my father had kept me alive through that grim time, we gave up most of our previous lifetime's arguments. I wouldn't choose to go about it the way I did, but depression allowed me to see love that had been there all along but had been obscure to me. I am therefore grateful not only to my father, but also to the sorrow he allayed.

the baby

ANNE LANDSMAN

I am the youngest of three, born eight years after my sister and five and a half years after my brother. As a child growing up in Worcester, a small town in South Africa, I was often referred to by my parents as a *laatlammetjie,* the last little lamb, the child that arrived well after the rest of the brood. On occasion, my mother still refers to me as her baby even though I have a daughter and a son of my own now, both no longer babies themselves.

I was acutely aware of being the youngest in the family, the last one to get potty-trained, the last one to lose a front tooth, the last one to learn to ride a bicycle, the last one to learn to read and write, the last one to grow breasts, graduate from high school, leave home. I was also the last one to get a job, get married, get a life. Being the youngest made me slow in some areas, and fast in others. It took me a long time before I learned the difference between left and right, before I felt comfortable in the kitchen, or handled my own money. I was always left behind in games of Monopoly, wondering to myself what mortgages were, baffled by the instructions on the back of the property cards.

But I also discovered that I was quick in school: I relished reading, writing, book-learning of all stripes. This is where I took the express rather than the local. At eight, I had already graduated to the grown-up section of the library, jostling old ladies for well-thumbed Regency romances, swallowing whole piles of books in one gulp. Throughout my childhood, I lived in a reading-induced stupor, moving in the real world like someone underwater. I was once even knocked down by a car while lost in my own thoughts. I was scolded by both parents for being a *loskop* (literally translated, a loose head), a daydreamer, a forgetter of things, slow to help out, both incompetent and disorganized. But just as often as they scolded me, they praised me for my high marks at school, my father describing me as "brrrilliant," rolling his *r*s with gusto. I was an idiot savant, witless but talented.

In 1976, my last year of high school, Soweto schoolchildren took to the streets, and riots rocked the country. During my years as an undergraduate at the University of Cape Town, I knew student leaders who had been banned, jailed, and deported for opposing the apartheid status quo. More camp-follower than activist, I attended rallies, listened to fiery speeches, and felt heartsick about my country. In 1981, I left for good, moving to New York City.

Fourteen years later, I was practically a New Yorker, having lived in many different parts of the city, from Inwood to Fort Greene. My favorite bus was the M104, the one that goes up and down Broadway. I was no longer the last one to learn things, but I still lived between the pages of a book. I had become a writer, had married James Wagman, an architect, and was pregnant with our first child. My brother lived in Rockville, Maryland, and had become a computational biologist at the National Institutes of Health. He was married, and his sons were five and eight. My sister lived in Wellesley, Massachusetts. She was a computer systems project manager at TJX Companies, was on to her second marriage, and had a son and a stepson, both teenagers. People often asked me—when they found out that my parents still lived in South Africa—why they hadn't moved to the United States since all their children and grandchildren were here. I could never answer them properly.

During the death throes of apartheid, when all hell was breaking loose, they never once considered leaving. Now, with a new South Africa in its infancy and Nelson Mandela at the helm, they were immensely grateful for the relatively smooth transition to democracy. Despite their advancing years, they were even less likely to leave. *Why was that?* I often wondered. *Was it money? Was it us? Was it them?* However, when I thought it over rationally, I knew the reason. My father was a country doctor in the heart of South Africa's wine region. My mother ran his practice. There was no comparable life for them in the United States, nothing to replace a lifetime of doctoring in the same small town. Where else but in this one corner of the world could my father say that he looked after four generations of one family? Where else could he find work, at seventy-five?

In addition to the economic and cultural reasons for them not leaving, there was also who we were as a family, the complex web of emotional forces that had led us to live such separate lives, an ocean and a continent between the children and the parents. We never were a warm and fuzzy family, largely because my parents were constantly arguing— sometimes little fights, sometimes big ones, and then all sizes in between. Even the good times had an edge to them, my mother raising an eyebrow sardonically, my father telling jokes at her expense. My mother was always the martyr, sighing dramatically, as she addressed my father with her oft-repeated line, "There you go again." And my father's responses to her provocations were often bloodcurdling, as he overturned chairs, lunged at her, drove his car wildly out of the driveway. She was forever criticizing him, controlling him, judging him. Because they worked together, she was privy to his every move, berating him for talking too much, eating too much, drinking too much. He was small, with a small man's rage at the world, and he responded to her dissatisfaction at his imperfections with force. On more than one occasion, he grabbed her around the neck, threatening to kill her.

Not surprisingly, they raised three fighters—my brother, my sister and myself—for whom angry bluster, a barbed retort, or a steely glare is much easier to muster than conciliatory words or openhearted gestures. There was—is—love between us but God forbid we should ever mention it, or show vulnerability of any kind. Vulnerability means sure death, and even today I can hear with perfect clarity the echoes of my father's curt "Buck up!" which he routinely said to us when we were upset, or my mother's "I'll give you something to cry about!"

In recent years, my mother has sometimes said, rather wistfully, after looking at old family photographs, "We're smiling in all the pictures. We were happy then, weren't we?" And yes, there were good times. I often felt, and still feel, close to my brother. There's one photo I especially cherish of him floating in the baby pool with me, when he'd long since outgrown being in such shallow water. There are pictures of us on holiday, my father

at the helm of his red-and-white boat, squinting into the sun with a look
of pride and pleasure on his face. There's a young, slim version of my
mother, laughing a big, open laugh and my sister, glamorous in a spotted
bathing suit, the midriff filled in with black netting. There are family trips
in the car, us eating homemade "Dagwood" sandwiches, pictures of family visiting from out of town, aunts in slacks, a short uncle with a sporty
beret on his bald head. Between border skirmishes, my parents laughed
at the same jokes, ate lots of chocolate, went to the movies every Friday
night after Shabbat dinner. Some nights, I could hear them murmuring in
bed, my room just across the hall from theirs. I would fall asleep, soothed
by the reassuring sound of them getting along. My mother, in one of her
warmer moments, confessed that she married my father because he made
her laugh. But, as the years progressed, the laughs seemed to diminish, and
their complaints about each other and about their failing bodies seemed
to grow.

They were always histrionic about their ailments, my father suffering
from a doctor's hypochondriacal sensitivity to the thousand and one ways
to have a terrible accident, a terrible disease, a terrible death. My mother,
working so closely with him for all those years and scarred, too, by witnessing her own mother's early death from breast cancer, was equally focused on her demise. Years ago, she sent a letter to her children in America
that opened with, "I do not have colon cancer." She then went on to describe how she thought she saw blood in her feces and had a colonoscopy
done. The letter is replete with an in-depth description of the procedure
as well as a small sketch of her colon. It turned out she'd eaten beets.

My father, whose father died from a pneumonia at forty-seven, began
to talk about his own death when he turned forty-seven. Every birthday
after that, it seemed, was going to be his last one. Weeks before the actual
day of his birth, August 14, he would begin to slide into a depression. His
somber mood would peak on or near his birthday, and then gradually lift
as the day receded into the past. Not only birthdays would bring on this
mood. A perceived slight from a colleague, a dark look from my mother, a
twinge in his back, a head cold, any number of injustices he felt the world
handed out to him would be causes for depression larded with rage. In
a lighter mood, he once handed out diagnoses for himself, my brother,

and me, as if passing on our birthrights. "I'm manic depressive!" he announced, in an excited voice. "And so are you," he continued, turning to my brother. "You are cyclothymic," he said to me, fixing me with his dark brown, slightly bulging eyes. On a good day, he could be riotously funny, his laughter infectious, his face wreathed in smiles. When something tickled him, he could laugh until he cried. But when his good humor evaporated—as it invariably did—he would become more and more gloomy, a storm cloud gradually settling over him and our home.

One year, when I must have been about ten, he came into my room in one of his black moods. I was home with a fever, sitting up in bed against the "big pillow," a special pillow brought out by my mother when we were sick. He was ferociously angry about something. He leaned over and hissed into my face, "I am going to kill myself one day!" I took him at his word, and began to live in terror that he was soon going to take his own life.

My childhood was full of fears about what my father might to do to himself, or to my mother. Just as he imagined the myriad ways he could die, I imagined, every time he stormed out of the front door after a fierce argument and marched across the street that separated our home from his office, that he was going to get a gun and shoot himself, or bring that gun into the house and shoot her. Living in apartheid South Africa mirrored the condition at home—barely suppressed violence constantly in the air, acts of rage bleeding into every aspect of life.

Leaving home, leaving the country was a huge relief. Like Woody Allen's gigantic, omnipresent mother floating in the sky in his short film, *Oedipus Wrecks,* my parents' heads seem to cover up the whole of South Africa on the map, obliterating everything else.

Finally, I could begin to breathe, to live. My relationship with my parents continued at a distance, the Sturm und Drang of our interactions muffled by the vast ocean between us, by the sometimes awkward phone connections, the time difference, and the growing cultural divide.

And then, in May 1995 my father—not my mother—was diagnosed with colon cancer. When the news came, I was eight months pregnant with my first child. Before my father's illness, there had been some talk of my mother coming to America for the birth of her first granddaughter.

Now that my father was sick and about to be operated on, she was staying by his side. Their constant bickering notwithstanding, they had always been there for each other, their marriage built as much on mutual dependency as resentment.

I couldn't help noting that my father, always one to share the minutiae of his bowel habits, to dwell on his fears about not getting to a toilet in time, was afflicted with a disease in the very area that had obsessed him his whole life. He was probably the worst candidate in the world for a colostomy bag, I thought, inwardly groaning. I began living with a new tension, worrying about the thing that I had always worried about finally coming to pass. There were many, many phone calls between us—me calling my parents in Worcester, calling my sister in Wellesley, calling my brother in Rockville. We were all in emergency mode, all of us with an edge in our voices, the love we could not express transformed into anger. Beneath our conversations, you could feel that there was a hunt for an enemy—someone was definitely, definitely to blame for this. I recall arguments about just how aggressive the cancer was, how operable, what the doctor in South Africa said or didn't say, what my mother said, or what my father said, who was right, who was wrong. And, in the irrefutable logic of family, we were all assigned to our various roles—the manager (my sister), the scientist (my brother), and the baby (me, of course).

In an effort to educate myself about the disease, I went to the Barnes & Noble on Astor Place and looked for a book on colon cancer. There are four stages of this disease and I had been told that my father had stage III. From the book, I learned that's one step removed from stage IV, the truly awful diagnosis where patients rarely live beyond five years. I zeroed in on the survival rate for Stage III sufferers—40 to 60 percent of them have a survival rate past five years. If I looked at the statistic one way, he was going to be seventy-six that year and a 40 to 60 percent chance of beating the odds and living to eighty-one didn't seem too bad. When I reversed it, giving him a 60:40 chance of dying, a cold hand clutched at my innards.

My brother mailed me my father's lab report, as well as two articles—one from the *Annals of Internal Medicine,* the other from the *Journal of Clinical Oncology*—about the chemotherapy treatment he would receive after his surgery. In the lab report, I got to see yet another sketch of one of my parents' colons, this one more professionally done. The "fungating" tumor measured 7 centimeters in diameter and the edges appeared "raised and lobulated." The sketch (of the mesocolon) was hard to decipher and looked like a very generalized map of Brooklyn.

My father was scheduled for surgery to remove the segment containing the tumor and reattach the colon. Thankfully, it seemed as if a colostomy would not be necessary. Post-surgery, he would begin chemotherapy with fluorouracil and levamisole. I scanned one of the articles my brother had sent me with its impressive title, "Fluorouracil plus Levamisole as Effective Adjudant Therapy after Resection of Stage III Colon Carcinoma." The scientific language washed over me. What was easier to remember was that these drugs were originally used to rid sheep, cows, and goats of internal parasites. My mind fixed on the image of sick sheep helping my father get better.

My sister was already making plans to fly to South Africa. She had a very concrete sense of what needed to be done. My brother was also talking about going there, perhaps after she left. As each day passed, the baby inside me grew. My due date was at the end of June, and it seemed to make little sense for me to make plans to go to South Africa, especially with my older siblings already en route. It was hard not to feel left out though, once again the baby sister pondering life's inscrutable instructions on the back of the Monopoly card. As a child, I had always had a horror of being left behind, while the older, bigger people took off somewhere without me. Trying to alleviate this feeling, I imagined the scenario at my father's bedside. There were no moments of grace, no loving gestures given or received. Love was the elephant in the room, the one thing no one was allowed to mention. I could hear my parents fighting though, with the occasional crackling laugh when my father made a wildly inappropriate joke or remark in front of the nurses, or exposed the site of his incision. I could imagine him making complicated attempts to use the toilet and talking about what he had or had not produced. Even from this distance, I could feel the embarrassment in the room, see my mother's irritation, watch my sister and brother pretend not to have heard.

When the surgery actually happened, there were some rough days that followed with pain and bowel difficulty of some kind. I was not close enough to know exactly what it was. I sent a dozen red roses and called as often as I could, focusing on how pleased he sounded when he heard my voice, how truly loved he seemed to feel those days, despite all our awkwardness with expressing it. When he shared some of the gory details, I immediately forgot them. After all, he couldn't show me where the surgeon opened him up. At this distance, his flapping hospital gown revealed nothing.

At the end of the year, my husband and I flew back to South Africa to see my parents with our six-month-old daughter, Tess, in tow. Mercifully, she slept in the bassinet clipped to the bulkhead for most of the seventeen-hour trip.

My father had had several months of chemotherapy by then. Amazingly, he looked every inch himself. Rotund (his suit size still a "portly short"), impish, every one of his luxuriant gray hairs in place. (Secretly, one of my worst fears was that my father would lose his thick shock of wavy hair.) Yes, he got tired after his treatments, extremely tired, but he still continued to see patients and seemed to have no intention whatsoever of retiring. Nothing had happened to his penchant for saying the preposterous, or his habit of drinking red wine. Like all my visits to South Africa, there were good times and bad times. My father had a tantrum in a restaurant overlooking the ocean, and my mother had one in a minivan on the way back from the Cango Caves. But they enjoyed their granddaughter immensely, my father paying me the peculiar compliment that I was a good mother of a small baby. I took in the glorious mountains, the minty air, and watched my delicious dandelion-puff of a daughter float in James's arms in a swimming pool, the same look of glee on her face that I remembered from the best days of my childhood, when the sun was hot and there was peace in our home.

Despite the bone-sapping exhaustion of his chemotherapy treatments, my father seemed euphoric at moments, buoyed by all the attention he'd been getting. I'd sent him *Love, Medicine and Miracles* to read after his surgery and now my father waved the book enthusiastically at me, claiming that he had learned something after all his years of doctoring—love actually does work magic.

We went back to South Africa again a year later. Tess was an eighteen-month-old toddler then, walking up a storm. She spent most of the plane ride walking up and down the aisles, walking and falling, walking, turning, falling down again. We were all zombies by the time we got off the plane.

This time, my father's mood was much darker. His optimism had dissolved, and he seemed tight-lipped, angry, depressed. With the cancer in remission, it appeared as if he had won the war but not the peace. A friend who had struggled with cancer explained that it was often easier to keep your spirits up when you were engaged with fighting the disease. It's the period after that can be most tricky, when the known enemy slips into the shadows, and you're faced with all the same problems that haunted you before you began your epic life-and-death struggle.

One afternoon we were having tea with my parents in their home, the same house I grew up in. The house is surrounded by a garden and borders a busy road. My father and Tess were sitting on the front *stoep*, Afrikaans for "porch." She was on his lap and he was reading to her from a board book.

Less than ten minutes later, my father came back into the house, into the room where James and I were having tea with my mother. "Where's Tess?" I asked. My father shrugged. I jumped up, shouting, "You were supposed to be looking after her!" My father responded, "She was supposed to be looking after me!" Ice in my veins, I raced outside, searching for my golden-haired child, imagining her walking through the garden gate into the traffic. Luckily, she was still on the *stoep*, which wrapped around the front of the house, and had walked down one side of it, instead of venturing down the steps toward the road.

This moment—with both generations battling each other for care—set me on edge. Relations with my father started to spiral down. I tried to recover, leaning on my patient, loving husband for support, staying close to my child.

I had recently sold my first novel, which was set in South Africa, and I was on the lookout while I was there for possible images for the cover. The novel took place in a town famous for its ostrich farms and underground cave system, the Cango Caves. My father had recently been given a collection of old photographs and old photographic negatives by a patient, who happened upon them at an estate sale. There were stacks and stacks of curling images in faded envelopes, the envelopes stuffed into brown boxes.

I started to go through the pictures, hoping to find something that might work. There was a heady excitement to the process, my joy at being published mixed with the thrill of the search. Finally, I struck gold—a turn-of-the-century image of a group of men and a lone woman in knee-length breeches standing in front of the entrance to the Cango Caves. They all held long candles in their hands, about to begin exploring.

I was practically delirious. The picture was uncannily perfect for my book. I searched through the box, finding the negative as well, which also seemed like a minor miracle. But my father didn't want to let the image out of his hands. He couldn't even consider the idea of my taking the negative and making a copy. In a stubbornly cruel maneuver, he took both the print and negative and locked them away in his room. My joy was now replaced by bitter disappointment, hurt, rage. That evening, as we were eating a rather miserable supper, I tried to cajole him into lending me the image. He looked at me, his eyes narrowing. "You're just like that girlie in *L.A. Law*," he said. "You'll do anything to get what you want."

I ran out of the house like an angry teenager. My mother tried to placate me. "I wish he were dead already!" I shrieked at her, my voice choked with pain. It felt like a curse.

By the time we left the following day, my mother had extracted the picture from him. He reluctantly handed over the brown envelope just before we got into the car to drive back to Cape Town.

Four months later, in April, we were celebrating Passover at our home in New York. I had just found out that I was pregnant with our second child. James and I hadn't told anybody yet. I got a phone call from South Africa. My mother told me that my father, after attending my uncle and aunt's golden wedding anniversary party in Cape Town, stepped off a curb the wrong way and fell down, breaking his arm. "It's a complicated fracture," she said, "a pathological fracture." My father got on the phone. "This is a bloody balls-up," he said ominously. "I don't think I'm going to make it this time." I could barely understand what he was trying to tell me. He was going to die from a broken arm? There was an awkward pause. I think he wanted me to reassure him, make him feel better. But I was tongue-tied. Perhaps he wanted me to say that I loved him, perhaps he wanted to say that he loved me. Perhaps he wanted to say that he was sorry for having acted so badly.

But we said none of these things. By the time I hung up, I was feeling a familiar cramping guilt. Somehow, it was my fault. I got through the evening in a haze of anxiety, the words "pathological fracture" ringing in my ears. What did it mean? I wondered.

I soon learned that it meant there was an underlying condition present making the bones more susceptible to fracture, and that the fracture had happened in a particularly awkward place. Apparently my father's self-diagnosed Paget's disease (a softening and weakening of the bone), which he believed he'd had for a while, is what had made the bone snap. I asked if it could be the cancer returning, but my question was brushed off with an ambiguous answer. No one wanted to consider that possibility seriously. Also, there was no clear person in charge, as my father had largely been his own doctor, and the usual records and history were absent. Since the surgery was going to be more difficult than the usual setting of a bone, some other options—leaving the arm alone or removing it—were discussed. My father wanted to keep working though, and undergoing the surgery was his best shot at having a usable hand.

Most of this information I gleaned in bits and pieces, mostly after the fact. During the actual surgery, I was on tenterhooks. Like all Landsmans, I had my own heightened fear of accidents, diseases, death. My husband, who comes from much more phlegmatic stock, tried to reassure me with "It's only a broken arm" and "Hasn't he cried 'wolf' many times before?"

I kept checking in with my mother that day, as she waited and waited for him to come out of surgery. The procedure took twice as long as expected. Hour after hour passed. Finally, he was moved into the nether-world of the recovery room. Here too, time stopped, and she had to wait for another long string of hours. When she finally saw him, she got the impression something hadn't gone as planned during the surgery. Initially, the doctors were going to give him a local block but something must have changed along the way and they put him to sleep using something called a laryngeal mask airway, a tube from the mouth down the throat, which rests against the larynx. He seemed extremely groggy, and since he was not breathing well enough on his own, the mask was still in place. His arm was bandaged up though, and that part of the operation seemed to have been a success. Later, an anesthesiologist cousin of mine visited him, and my father sat up and talked to him.

Things did not go well in the night and my father was taken to a hospital with an ICU in Paarl, the town where the anesthesiologist lived. Things were grouping themselves erratically in my imagination. There were two anesthesiologists—the cousin visiting from Texas and the man who put him under, who seemed to be in charge of my father's care—and two medical facilities, the nursing home in Cape Town, where he was operated on, which had no ICU, and the hospital in Paarl, where he was now, which had an ICU. Years later, I would parse this information and wonder why events unfolded the way they did. But then we were in the thick of it; my father's lungs had filled with fluid, and he was struggling to breathe.

I spoke to the anesthesiologist, Dr. Boezaart, who felt that although this was a setback, my father would pull through. In the meantime, my sister flew to South Africa. Within days, I got a fax from her relating that my father had continued to have problems getting the phlegm up from his lungs and that the doctor had performed a tracheotomy to relieve his breathing.

He was on a respirator, and the next few days were rocky. He fought with the nurses when they tried to keep all the tubes in, and they eventually had to strap him down. In the midst of this, my mother told him that I was pregnant, and he responded by enthusiastically rattling all the equipment that he was attached to. Soon after, he was off the respirator and able to communicate by writing things down on a scrap of paper. When I asked the nurse to ask him how he was feeling, he wrote down, "social, comfortable, and improving," as if he was doing a ward-round and was making observations about one of his own patients. Although he could breathe on his own now, his kidney function had slowed to a halt. On the phone, Dr. Boezaart recited numbers to me. If the low numbers climb higher, he said, my father would make it. The numbers didn't move.

My father slid into a coma induced by end-stage renal failure. There was little talk of dialysis, my mother telling us that he wouldn't have wanted it. My brother left for South Africa.

I had to make a decision about whether or not I was going to go, too, as it became clear that nothing short of a miracle would save my father's life. My brother arrived and called me after visiting our father. He was crying over the phone, a high-pitched keening sound, the saddest cry I had ever heard. "He's so still," he said finally.

As my father lay dying in his hospital bed, I was acutely aware of the new life quickening inside me. I was unusually tired, and tried to rest. Whenever grief at my father's plight raged through my system, I tried to calm myself, breathe deeply. It took James and me nearly eighteen months to conceive our first child. Now, two and half years later, I was thirty-eight and even more aware of the fragility and preciousness of this pregnancy.

I called my ob/gyn to ask whether flying to South Africa would endanger the fetus. She focused on what concerned me the most. "It's not the flight per se that's the problem," she explained. "It's the stress of what you might encounter there. How that might or might not affect you is what's hard to predict." Also, the fertilized egg had so recently embedded itself that it was more easily dislodged at this early stage than later. "Still," she concluded, "I would not tell you not to go. It's something only you can decide."

Walking the city streets, when I looked at the faces of women roughly my age, all I could think was, *What would they do in my position? What about that blond woman reading on the subway, would she risk losing a child to see her father before he dies? Or the woman behind the counter at our local deli, would she go?*

I always returned to the scenario of me actually getting on a plane and flying to Cape Town. When I arrive, my mother is all over me with her concern for my condition, and I'm suddenly the baby again, suffocatingly so. She's telling me I'm eating too little, I look exhausted, I have to rest. She's inches from my face, breathing on me. When I try to protest, she gets furious, deeply hurt. My sister's in hypercompetent mode, organizing everything, telling everyone what to do. Here, too, I am the baby again as she bosses me around. My brother's numb and mostly silent

until he disagrees with something. Then he digs in his heels and fights to
the death like the rest of us. There aren't too many warm hugs or kind
words exchanged, not too much of "I know how you feel, and I feel it,
too." There's an unspoken competition for who has the right information,
who's doing the most, who's suffering the most.

Perhaps this was an extremely ungenerous portrait of my family, but
at that moment I couldn't imagine getting off the plane, jet-lagged and
grief-stricken, and anyone being nice to me.

If it weren't for the tiny life I was carrying, I would have weathered
the abrasiveness, the bluster with which we covered up our vulnerabili-
ties, the inevitable moments of discord—all the particular ways, to paraphrase the first sentences of *Anna Karenina,* this family was unhappy. But
then it seemed like an impossible task.

Although my sister didn't say it, I got the impression that she thought
I should be at my father's bedside. She was full of stories about what she
was doing and how difficult it was, and there was always the unspoken
memory of the last time, when my father had colorectal surgery and I
was missing, too. Though my brother diplomatically declined to have an
opinion on whether I should go or not, I would have liked to have been
there with him, sharing his pain and grief at closer quarters. My mother,
to her great credit, didn't put any pressure on me at all, telling me to do
what was best for me, and for the baby.

I spoke to the doctor in South Africa to get yet another point of view.
He asked me to consider what my doctor-father would have advised, had
he been conscious. The answer was clear. He would have said "Choose
life." Even if the odds were great that nothing bad would have happened,
why take any risk at all?

Still, as I came closer and closer to deciding not to go, it was impossible for me to feel any peace or closure. I couldn't get away from the
image of my father in his hospital bed, his craggy face in profile—beaked
nose, small, sardonic mouth, twinkling eyes forever closed. Help came
from a Jesuit priest, Father Ed, whom my in-laws had met on a recent trip
to Ireland. Father Ed recommended that I write a letter to my father and
have a family member read it to him.

I sat down to write, remembering what made my father's character so vivid, so alive. He loved fruit, and watching him peel and eat an orange always made you want to eat one yourself. He was passionate about the town he grew up in, as well as the little seaside resort nearby where he had summered since he was a child. Through him, I'd learned about neap tides and spring tides, the habits of bluebottles, the pleasures of boating on a meandering river that started in the mountains and emptied itself into the sea. His greatest passion of all was his love of doctoring. I remembered him coming home after having delivered a baby, blood spots on his white shirt, his tie, joyfully proclaiming, "It's a boy!" or "It's a girl!" Tears streaming down my cheeks, I wished him well on this mysterious journey he was about to undertake, and I told him how much I loved him.

The letter was faxed to South Africa and read to my father, who lay motionless in his bed. Within days, he was dead. As my siblings and my mother organized his funeral, I remained in New York. I couldn't help them in any way because I was here, the baby carrying her own baby. It was hard not to feel incompetent, helpless, the *loskop laatlammetjie* all over again. On the other side of the world, my father had a big funeral, and our house in Worcester was choked with people of all colors, races, and backgrounds coming to pay tribute to the little doctor who had cared for them all so well. In New York, I arranged for prayers at our home, and a rabbinic intern from my synagogue officiated. As I intoned the kaddish, the sun drained out of the sky, its last rays lighting up the Twin Towers visible from our front windows.

I was stunned at how bereft I felt, even though there were so many miles separating my father and myself, so many years of distance, so much childhood hurt. I felt cold all the time, as if I was about to get sick. I began to understand the animal nature of grief, the mourning of dogs, apes, elephants. The loss of my father was huge, as if someone had taken off a limb. Not only had I lost him, the idiosyncratic, lovable rascal that he was, I had also lost a fantasy. When he was alive, there was always the hope that he would turn one day into a real father, the benign, openhearted father I dreamed of having. Now that dream was gone, too.

Months passed in a blur. That September when I went to synagogue on Yom Kippur, a vision of my father appeared to me during the Yizkor service, a memorial service for the dead. He was wearing a yarmulke on his head and had a prayer shawl around his shoulders. He was smiling at me, the warmest smile in the world, and his eyes were twinkling as if he was very happy to see me there. Three months later my son, Adam Gabriel Wagman, was born. The *g* of his second name is for Gerald, my father's name. In Hebrew, he is Yakov Baruch, just like my father.

Now, when I look into my son's chocolate-brown eyes, dark and light at the same time, my father winks back at me, so glad I chose life.

death in slow motion

ELEANOR COONEY

My mother was always my favorite person. Hip, cool, brilliant, funny, sane. A writer. Mary Durant. I have a picture of her from one summer in the mid-1960s in the backyard of our house in Connecticut. She's in the midst of me and a bunch of my teen-aged friends, sitting in a canvas chair, slim, elegant blue-jeaned legs crossed, laughing. We're all free and easy, horsing around, performing for her. She's in her early forties, beautiful, probably a year or so away from meeting Mike, her third husband, the love of her life. When they married in 1966, he was thirty-two and she was forty-four.

Whoever it was who said love is stronger than death was full of ma-larkey. When Mike died in 1989, my mother's own life was pretty much sucked out of her. It will get easier eventually, everyone said, but it didn't. It got worse. She rallied for a while—took a job as curator of the local his-torical museum and even wrote another book. But her heart was shred-ded. I could always hear it in her voice when she answered the phone. The first shadows fell around 1997, with blanks in her short-term memory and uncharacteristic lapses in judgment. She was seventy-five years old at the time, and I have no doubt that protracted despair had plenty to do with her mental deterioration. My theory is that it affected the physical structure of her brain, softened it, made her vulnerable to the disease. She's graduated to delusions and disorientation and now some long-term memory loss, too. My mother was truly gorgeous once—wavy brown hair, brown-green eyes full of wit and intelligence, an aquiline nose with a classy hump in it, a sexy gap between her two front teeth—and she aged well, tall and trim. Time, grief, and dementia have bent her a little, but she's still a handsome woman, her speech and demeanor surprisingly normal. If you didn't know her before and you met her briefly, you might not notice anything wrong. If you were someone who knew her well, the change you'd see first is in her eyes: they're alert, but blank and dead at the same time.

In September 1998 my brother and I and my mate, Mitch, went to Connecticut and began the process of ripping my mother up by the roots and moving her to California. We had to. Her old friends were calling, telling us things weren't right at all, that she was confused, bursting into tears, forgetting the way to peoples' houses that she'd been going to for decades, denting up her car, repeating questions five times during one phone conversation, then calling up and asking the same questions again, drinking too much, obsessively mourning Mike, getting hoodwinked out of thousands of dollars by phony sweepstakes telemarketers. She's only going to get worse, my brother said. We can't just sit and wait for disaster. We have to get her out now. One more winter alone there and something really bad will happen.

I would never have had the courage to make such a decision, but he did. It looks to me like Alzheimer's, he said.

He may as well have suggested elephantiasis. Not possible, I said. Not her. All our ancient relatives kept their marbles right up to the end. She's just depressed or something. It couldn't be Alzheimer's.

But then I remembered a small, uneasy moment I'd relegated to some uninhabited corner of my mind and experienced a nasty and prescient little squirt of adrenaline recollecting it: My mother, on a recent visit to California, standing in front of my house looking at my car, a peculiar, baffled, scared expression in her eyes. "Where's *my* car?" she said. Her car, of course, was nearly three thousand miles away, in Connecticut.

I had for years entertained a fond but hazy vision of my mother eventually moving out to California to live near me. We'd have fun. We'd be together. Especially since Mike's death, I was always sorry about the vast continent between us and all the time that went by without seeing each other. Now the move was on us, abruptly and unceremoniously, and I felt like a monster. She alternated between compliance and cooperation and crying and screaming. But I knew that once we got her settled in my own little idyllic Northern California seaside town that I'd be able to help her. We'd found her a beautiful small apartment a block from my house, sent things ahead to decorate the place and make it homey—books, pictures, a few choice pieces of furniture, and most important, her trusty old manual typewriter—and packed up the rest for sale in Connecticut by a couple of auctioneers. No more worries, Mom, we said. Now you can write your memoirs.

She'd stay in Connecticut for the month of October. Mitch and I would go out to California and prepare. We'd make her happy. No more dinners alone, lots of loving attention, vitamins, therapy. I'd restore her faltering memory. I'd find a way to solve her mysterious chronic upset stomach. Give her a new life.

She arrived on schedule at the end of October. An old friend had come up from New York and spent the final week with her, helping her pack, making sure she stuck to the plan. Then Mike's best friend escorted her and Polly, her cat, out to the airplane. Everything was ready.

She got a new life, all right, and so did we. Within a scant two months of my mother's arrival, I find myself hiding in the dark about forty feet from the sliding glass door of the kitchen. My heart is pounding with fury, sorrow, anguish. Light casts itself partway across the yard, but I imagine looking out from the inside and know Mitch won't be able to see me. A few minutes before, he did what men allow themselves to do: stomped out in a rage and slammed the door. We'd had a huge fight because I hadn't got my mother out of there and back to her apartment with enough dispatch after dinner. I'll be fucked, I thought, if I'll just sit in the house and wait like a woman for him to come back. When he does, I won't be here. He can wonder where I am. And I'll find a place where I can spy on him. I'll wait, even if it takes three hours, and I'll watch him when he doesn't know he's being watched. I want to see him look for me. And then I'll make *him* wait.

Stability and predictability in daily routine are what the sages prescribe for people with Alzheimer's. They have wise words for the caregivers: Take care of yourself. Give yourself a break. Be sure to set aside time to do the things you enjoy. Get plenty of rest. Pamper yourself. Enlist the help of friends and relatives to assist with your loved one. Take time out for yourself, they chant. Time out for yourself? I'll let you in on a secret. There is no time out, not even when you are sound asleep, if the person is in fact a loved one and money is scarce.

Money. It can't buy back a person's mind, but it can go a long way toward helping you save your own. My mother arrived with some monthly income. Mitch and I are both writers, which means that we sometimes have to do other things to pay the bills. I was under contract to write a novel about eighth-century China (indentured, I should say, because the manuscript was way overdue and the advance by then a dim memory). The time when Mitch would have been doing other things to support the household had to go to my mother's care and attention. In our perfect naïveté we had not anticipated just how much care and attention that would be. Before we knew it, we were financially dependent on her.

And then there was plenty of good old-fashioned guilt: guilt over dragging my mother away from her home, guilt over what I was inflicting on Mitch. He'd been a single father and had raised three children from diapers to adulthood. He'd more than earned his freedom, and now, because of me, he was in a domestic trap again. This is not fair, I thought. This was not what he signed on for. We weren't even officially married; he was under no obligation to stay.

"I'll do this," he said at the beginning, "but I can't promise I'll always be nice."

I knew he wouldn't quit or walk away. The fact that he'd raised children meant he was far better prepared for what we'd taken on than I, who'd assiduously avoided parenthood because I'd never wanted the responsibility. It was both reassuring and alarming to know he was in it for the duration. His jaw was clenched after only a week or so of having my mother around, and we were looking at infinity. Although we were still like the proverbial blind men feeling an elephant in the dark, we were starting to get an idea of the size and shape of the creature called Alzheimer's.

And it wasn't as if she had forced herself on us. She had begged to be allowed to stay in Connecticut. But we'd brought her, and it was my responsibility to make her happy. What have we done? whispered the voice of doom when my eyes popped open at dawn shortly after her arrival. *What have we done?*

I clung fast to my optimistic visions. We took her to a good doctor for a complete physical. He put her on antidepressants. A psychologist tested her thoroughly and diagnosed her with "probable" Alzheimer's. They don't know what causes it—the theories range from aluminum pots to an autoimmune disorder—but the prognosis is irreversible memory loss and disorientation until you don't recognize your children, your husband, your wife, the process slower in some people than in others, and eventually you forget to eat, swallow, breathe. Not all dementia is Alzheimer's, and a definitive diagnosis can be made only postmortem, with microscopic examination of brain tissue. Most cases of dementia, though, *are* Alzheimer's, I was told. But I was not ready to consign my mother to the bone heap. Even if it was Alzheimer's, I'd beat it.

I ordered special brain nutrients off the Internet. Mitch made a trip to Tijuana to get more. He also discovered that my mother was putting away formidable amounts of vodka. He marked her bottle and found that during the night its contents dropped by a full two measuring cups. My mother weighs about 125 pounds. The effect on her of a couple of martinis was truly scary, as if she'd been punched in the head. One night shortly after she got to California, we went out to dinner. We had drinks. During the dinner, she asked whether we were in Southbury or New Milford, towns in Connecticut. Afterward, we went to the all-night Safeway, and my mother stood there under the fluorescent lights with real terror on her face and, her voice weirdly even, said: "I don't have the slightest idea where I am or why."

She'd always been a controlled, moderate cocktail drinker. Never when I was growing up did I see her even a little tipsy, and she was utterly disdainful of sloppy drunks. She still insisted she never drank more than a couple of martinis a day, and only at dinnertime. It wasn't that she was lying or covering up. It was that she couldn't remember.

Mitch's theory, that her memory loss was booze-induced, was exciting. God, we thought, maybe we can get my mother back just by sobering her up. And maybe sobering her up will fix everything else, too! For about three years, she'd been complaining of a queasy stomach, shakiness, feeling generally lousy. She'd been to gastroenterologists from one end of Connecticut to the other, and they could find nothing wrong. Vodka, she claimed, settled her stomach—thus the daytime and late-night swigging. But now we believed liquor might be the culprit in her gastric distress as well as her memory loss.

So we took her off the hard stuff completely and gave her ersatz wine instead. We made a ceremony of it: ice cubes clinking cheerily and suggestively at the "cocktail hour." We knew it might take some time to see real results, but now we had something tangible to work with.

And every night, when I escorted her back to her apartment, I laid out her vitamins, supplements, brain nutrients, herbal stomach soothers, antidepressant, digestive enzymes.

Our hopes were high. Looking back, I can't even remember what that felt like. It was gradual possession: this person looked like my mother, sounded like my mother, but she was becoming everything that had been anathema to her: intrusive, complaining, hypochondriacal. And that thing that most of us would rather die than be, designated by Oscar Wilde as the only valid criterion by which one divides up the human race, the condition she would have dreaded most of all: tedious.

The friends and good times I had envisioned did not materialize. At first, I worked hard to introduce her to people. Tragic factors quickly became evident: When I did introduce her to someone, she forgot that person instantly. A long, fun dinner party would evaporate from her memory before we'd said the last good night. What's the point of fun if you can't remember it? And the sad truth is that when people catch a whiff of dementia, they back off quickly. When the party's over, they don't call back. Who can blame them?

That was particularly hard for me to watch. This was a woman who had been social all her life. Her charm and manners were hard-wired into her so thoroughly that she could still pull it together most of the time and fool people for a while. For a while. Then she'd slip, repeat something she'd just said, or maybe say something odd about being in Connecticut, and I'd see the little moment of comprehension on peoples' faces.

A deep streak of contrariness in my mother also helped to nullify my efforts. Mitch was acting in a local play that winter. My mother often talked about joining the theater group. She'd been onstage a lot in her day, a member of Actor's Equity. She'd been damned good. I'd like to try out, she said. Mitch and I zipped our lips at the notion of a woman with Alzheimer's learning lines—indeed, even remembering that she was in a play—but I took her to one of his rehearsals, thinking that maybe she could help the actors practice their lines, or make friends, or just be entertained. She sat for about fifteen minutes and then whispered that she was bored and wanted to go home.

If I took her to an informal session of singing (she used to love to sing) at a local musician's house, she'd sit, silent and diffident, then whisper that she felt lousy and wanted to go home. And writing? Forget it. My mother's prolific typewriter had always thundered away up on the top floor of the house in Connecticut. Now it sat silent and dusty. She didn't like the action of the keys, she said (never mind that it was her own machine). So I got her another. And another. Soon she had four typewriters lined up on her desk. Plenty of paper, pencils, Wite-Out. The only thing I ever saw her write was half a letter, never finished, and the effort cost her a week of fretting and fluttering. Now *that* really scared me.

A terrible transformation began to take place in me as well: This mother I had once loved to show off because she was so much cooler and smarter than anyone else's mother now embarrassed me. I scrambled to cover up the gaps, to compensate, and before long, to hide her.

How quickly our own little prison clanged shut around the three of us. Our lives became a hellish ritual: My daily phone call to her, 9:00 A.M. sharp. Mitch delivering the morning paper to her, visiting with her to keep her away from me for a while so I could try to get some work done in the morning. Her sighs of desolation and loneliness. Her yearning to return to Connecticut and the vanished good times. Both of us trying to explain why that wasn't possible. Tears over Mike, as fresh and hot as if he had died just yesterday. My churning, muddy emotions while I desperately tried to write about plague and murder in Canton in A.D. 750, at triple speed.

Afternoons, a kindly fellow we hired, though we couldn't afford it, took her out in our car and tried to keep her diverted until the dinner hour and her appearance at our door. She was still making her own breakfast and lunch, but dinner alone was unthinkable. There had been way too many lonely dinners with too much vodka in Connecticut. I had pledged that there would be no more lonely nights, but I had envisioned friends and activities. . . .

I had also envisioned her strolling to the market a few blocks away in our beautiful town, doing some of her shopping for herself. Forget that, too. She had a hard time finding her way from her apartment to our house, though she could sure as hell find her way to the liquor store at the other end of town, and even talk them into taking her Connecticut check. Which meant we had to keep her wallet empty and her checkbook and credit card away from her if she was going to spend any time at all alone at her apartment so that *we* could have some time alone at our house. And purloining her checkbook and credit card and keeping her wallet empty meant that we had to do a lot of fast-talking and fancy footwork and all of her shopping for her. We had to control her, exert discipline on her, fib and dissemble, all of it perfectly contrary to how I was accustomed all my life to relating to my mother. It affected me the way it would if someone held a gun to my head and told me I had to skin cats or be an airline stewardess. I hated it, but I had no choice. Luckily for me, Mitch had resolve where I did not.

We were all that stood between her and aloneness. So: Dinner each and every evening, on time, at our house. My efforts to keep her occupied and entertained and out of Mitch's hair. Her repertoire of conversational topics—stories from the past we could have recited in unison with her, or how much she missed Mike and why did he have to die and how she wished she could just die herself. My own sorrow over Mike dredged up and renewed. Then the requests for vodka, the explanations of why she couldn't have it, the amazing perpetual-staircase conversations:

"Is there any hard liquor in the house?"

"No, Mom. No hard liquor. Doctor's orders."

"I don't see what difference it makes at my age. And it settles my stomach."

"It messes up your head. You don't know where you are or who you are. Besides, we've been told"—lie—"that hard liquor is a dangerous mix with your antidepressants."

"Oh?"

"Yes. Very bad. And you want to get your memory back, don't you?"

"Of course I do."

"So let's try an experiment. No hard liquor for a while."

"All right. I'm willing to give it a try."

"Good! Here's some wine."

"Is there any hard liquor in the house?"

And every night, dinner on little folding tables in front of the television. CNN, *Jeopardy!*, *Win Ben Stein's Money*. We were shunted into that routine quickly; she wanted it, it diverted her, we felt compelled to defer to her, and of course we couldn't just let her sit there by herself, so we joined her. And there we were, as if we'd been doing it for a thousand years, and would be doing it for another thousand.

Then came one of the saddest and cruelest developments of all. The one thing that brought her a bit of contentment, the thing she'd wanted so much since Mike's death, to be a member of a household and family again, became a source of acute irritation to both Mitch and me: My mother, happily bumbling around the kitchen, clattering dishes, opening and shutting cupboards and drawers over and over again because she couldn't remember where anything was, trying to put things away or to set out the silverware. Bumping into us, standing right behind us while we cooked, her cigarette smoke curling around our eyes and noses.

The evenings ended with me walking her home, laying out her vitamins, cleaning her cat box. Running the tub for her while she objected like a little child.

"But I took a bath this morning!"

Here's an intimate and unhappy fact of senile dementia: They become unappetizing. They don't bathe unless you make them. They'll wear dirty underwear and never wash their hair. Their fingernails and feet will be grimy. Unclean children are one thing; unclean old people are quite another. You will begin to find a person you love . . . odious. And you will hate yourself for feeling it.

And after the bath, the bedtime merry-go-round conversations:

"Who are the women who are taking things out of my house?"

"No one's taking anything out of your house, Mom. Everything's safe and sound."

"Someone called me and said two women were emptying my house and putting everything in storage."

"Nope. No women are taking anything out of your house. If they were, I'd know about it. You have a house sitter. Everything's fine."

"What's my house sitter's name?"

"Billy Reynolds."

"Ah, yes. Billy Reynolds. And he's taking care of things?"

"Yep. And doing a great job."

"I'll have to go back and empty the house."

"It's mostly done, Mom. Remember? We were all there together in the fall."

"But there are books and pictures and things I want to go through."

"It's mostly done. We'll go back when the house sells."

"But I should empty it out before it sells."

"That's not necessary. Selling a house isn't like selling a car. They don't just write a check and move in the next day. There's plenty of time."

"But who are the women who are taking things out of my house?"

Having a parent with dementia in your household means that everything (and I mean everything) in your life immediately arranges itself around the dementia. It's like having a two-year-old, but with some obvious and important differences. The process of the child becoming the parent, which is of course what happens, was bitter confusion for me. She'd been my mother, so accomplished, so generous, so polite, so kind to me, always so lucid and sensible, that my wish to defer to her and please her and impress her—and most of all, not to lose her—only very slowly and with the most stubborn reluctance gave way to the unwelcome knowledge that I was now Mommy. And a not very good one. A snappish, desperate, incompetent Mommy.

When it was just us, Mitch and I ran a fairly routine-free household. We'd eat together, or he'd eat when he felt like it and I'd eat when I felt like it. After my mother's arrival we produced 558 dinners, on schedule, every night, without fail—probably 557 of them in front of the TV.

And every day, without fail, she'd ask: "Am I having dinner with you tonight?" Or, a slight variation, spoken in a piteous voice that caused both me and Mitch to grind our teeth: "Is there enough food for me to eat with you tonight?" Pretty lousy acting, Mitch observed.

Sarcasm rose to my tongue. Sometimes I could check it. Sometimes I couldn't. "No, Mom," I'd say. "There's not enough food. You're going to eat cold gruel tonight, alone, in the dark."

Moneylessness, my manuscript deadline, guilt, sorrow, relentless responsibility, and no life of our own: we were trapped, swimming hopelessly in circles, sinking, hearing my mother's ever-narrowing set of refrains, recited daily like the stations of the cross, each one a knife in my heart: her homesickness, her loneliness, missing Mike, and the one that made us craziest of all—her stomach. Oh, God. Her stomach.

The doctors and hospitals she'd gone to all over Connecticut gave her every test known to medical science. No one could find anything wrong, but she was in misery. One gastroenterologist I talked to on the phone when we were moving her out of her house spoke sharply of how she had got hold of his home number and called him there, more than once. I apologized. "You realize that your mother is suffering from dementia, don't you?" he said without sympathy. "Uh, yes," I said, but of course I had no notion at all then of the real meaning of the ugly word.

She'd complain of nausea and "seasickness" almost every day. It didn't take long for us to see that abstinence from liquor not only was failing to restore her memory but was having no effect whatsoever on her stomach. So we took her to doctors, acupuncturists, chiropractors. Mitch drove her hundreds of miles to specialists. She had prescription medicines, she had Chinese herbal medicines, she had bitter witch's-brew herbal concoctions that we made in the pressure cooker. Sometimes we had a few days' respite and thought we'd found the cure, but always, always, it came roaring back. Sometimes there were acute attacks when she'd cry and tremble and double over with pain. I admit I caved in a couple of times and let her have a drink, but it did nothing at all for her stomach, and even a small drink magnified her brain damage in a way that was anything but fun or soothing for her and was alarming as hell for me.

Mitch and I argued. He believed that some of the time her pain was real, but that there were other times when she faked it—not necessarily consciously but reflexively, he theorized—to get my attention and sympathy, to get a drink. I said maybe, it sure seems that way sometimes, but what if it *is* real? I can't afford *not* to believe it's real. Imagine yourself senile, I said, and suffering, and everyone around you sick of hearing about it and ignoring you. It's a thought not to be borne.

And of course, I *was* getting sick of hearing about it. Her complaints, her face gray with pain, her confusion, her questions about doctors, hospitals, and pharmacists—repeated verbatim virtually every day as if we'd never discussed the topic before—became torture for us all. She'd groan, stagger, weep, hold her stomach. As the months progressed, and nothing we tried worked, I came to live in a chronic state of rage and helplessness—rage at my failure, helplessness in the face of this infuriating, baffling stomach demon that wrecked any chance at all of making my mother's life even a little bit pleasanter. It was bad enough that she had to lose her mind; it was intolerable that she should also suffer physically almost all the time, that nothing could be done, that she couldn't understand or remember how hard we'd tried, that even the kindest doctors didn't want to hear about it anymore, that Mitch and I got so raw with impatience that we could barely stand to hear another word about it. It was a nattering nightmare. Don't take it out on her, don't take it out on her, I rebuked myself. Don't.

But sometimes I did. Not that I beat her or anything crude like that. I promise I didn't. I mostly succeeded at being patient. I wanted more than anything to relieve her pain, but there were times when I snapped at her, yelled, stamped my foot or clenched my fists and hissed with poisonous exasperation. Mitch, my valiant trouper most of the time, raised his voice more than once. She'd cry. "I wish I could just die," she'd say. "If I had a gun I'd shoot myself."

Then came remorse and more self-flagellation. Was this what my mother deserved, in her sickness and loss? To be at the mercy of a couple of ill-tempered louts like us? Had I really tried everything to help her, or was I just giving up because I'm too selfish and stupid and lazy to find the cure? She, who would always come to my rescue. I felt hard and mean and full of sorrow all at once, and it drove me truly mad. Drove me, in fact, to drink.

When we first told her she'd have to stay off the vodka, we were honorable. If we were going to ask her to abstain, then so would we. Such integrity! In just a couple of months, we were the ones with hidden bottles. We moved like sorcerers, deftly bringing out the hooch while she was right there in the room with us and her attention was diverted for a moment, pouring ourselves stiff ones and drinking them nonchalantly out of coffee cups right in front of her. Sometimes in the middle of the day. Sometimes in the morning, something I'd never done in my life.

I discovered a wee shot at dawn to be the best way to shut down my poor roiling head and get back to sleep for another hour or two. I found Zen-like little oases of peace and solitude, propped on my pillow and staring into my soft red night-light at 6:00 A.M., sipping from a cup, feeling the alcohol spread subtly from my stomach to my limbs and brain, displacing the residue from disturbing dreams. Like this one: I'm at my mother's house in Connecticut. Mike has come back to life for a while, just a while, we all know it's only temporary, and he and my mother are stripping the house bare, even taking down the walls.

Connecticut. Her wit, her intellect, her creativity all erode away like desert sandstone while Connecticut stands solid in her memory.

"I think I'll go back to Connecticut and live with Joan Talbridge."

"Mom, you can't go live with Joan Talbridge."

"Why not?"

"Because she has a life of her own. She can't take care of you. She's not your family."

"I don't think I need to be taken care of."

"But you do. Your memory's full of holes. You need to be with your family."

"Joan invited me to come live with her."

"She invited you for a visit. Not to live with her. To visit. She can't do the job that a family does."

"Give me some examples of some of these goofy things I'm supposed to have done."

"Well, the fact that we've already had this conversation about fifty times is one example."

"No, really. Give me some examples."

"Well, you were bilked out of almost eight grand. You couldn't find your way to old friends' houses where you'd been going for forty years. You were depressed and crying whenever I called you on the phone. You called me once to say you'd taken Polly to a kennel, but you couldn't re-member which one, so you called all of them and none of them had her, and then it turned out Polly was shut in the basement. Every one of your old friends was worried about you. They called me and Timmy up to tell us they were worried about you."

"They were worried about me?"

"Yes. All of them. Because of little things that were adding up. Joan Talbridge was one of the people who was worried about you."

"Give me some examples."

"I just did. That's an example."

"I could go live with Joan Talbridge."

April 1999: We were moving. We'd decided it would be easier on us and on her to have her on the same property but in her own little house. Far from the liquor store. As it was, we were running back and forth between her apartment and our rented house ten times a day, and when I was at my house I could feel the force field of her loneliness emanating from the direction of her apartment like a tractor beam.

There was a gap of about a month between the time when the lease on my mother's apartment would be up and the time when we'd be able to move her into the new house (my brother arranging the incredibly complicated financing from afar). So we had to move her out of the apartment, pack all her stuff, scrub and clean the place so we'd get the deposit back, and temporarily stash her in the run-down little studio in the backyard of the old house—all in the midst of packing up our own life detritus, tossing it feverishly into boxes like fleeing refugees, stuffing it into the car, and taking it up to the new house, trip after trip after trip.

I was still struggling with my manuscript, three more chapters to go, so Mitch had to do most of the packing. I'd sit at my computer in my ransacked study and write for a few hours every day while he tramped nonstop past my door carrying furniture and huge boxes and my mother wandered in and out, her confusion multiplying exponentially, no idea at all what we were doing or why, presenting me with tattered grocery lists from months before.

We moved the washer and dryer, cages of yowling cats (ten—yeah, I know), dressers that fell off trucks, scattering socks and underwear in the street. We stayed up until 4:00 A.M. three nights in a row cleaning and scrubbing the old house. Then we moved my mother into the master bedroom of the new house while Mitch and I, a couple of stumbling zombies, burrowed in among piles of books and clothing in the spare room. Meanwhile, a carpenter was converting the garage into a "granny unit" for my mother, my brother again handling the financing. As soon as that unit is finished, we told ourselves, everything will be fine. No more running back and forth between house and apartment in town. She'll be snug in her own little place and we'll be just a few steps away.

One evening shortly after we moved in, Mitch made a little joke to my mother about "room service" when he brought her a snack on a tray. She laughed, accepted the snack, and pretended to tip him. Aha, I thought—a little moment of normalcy. I was pathetically grateful.

The next morning, she was dressed and sitting on the window seat in the living room.

"There's no need to stay here any longer," she said. "We should check out now."

I was barefoot, in my bathrobe, hair mashed, a Breathe Right stuck to my nose.

"Where," I asked cautiously, "do you think we are?"

I saw a flash of fear in her eyes.

"Isn't this a hotel?"

The independence we envisioned for her and the end to her awful loneliness because she'd have her own cozy little house a mere ten feet away from ours turned out to be our worst delusion so far. She became our prisoner, and we became hers, in a way that made the endless winter before we moved seem like a tea party.

She lived in the house with us for about six weeks before the cottage was finished enough for us to move her in. This house has a great big kitchen and dozens of cupboards. Her cupboard-banging back in the kitchen at the old house, searching for utensils whose location she could never learn, had annoyed us, but now she was like a musician going from a small electronic keyboard to a mighty church organ. There are thirty-six cupboard doors in the kitchen, each with a slightly different pitch. Mitch and I lay in bed in our junk-packed little room at dawn or the middle of the night listening to the symphony: BANGETY-BANG BANG BANG! BANG! BANGETY-BANG!

This banging was a sound wired into my system from as far back as my childhood. When she was young and whole, my mother had had an impressive temper, and cupboard noise was one of its expressions. Now, in 1999, every BANG sent shock waves of mingled associations, one ancient and primal and the other very recently acquired, along my worn and frazzled nerves directly to my brain. It was around then that I noticed myself getting seriously jumpy. I flinched and twitched and leapt at any small unanticipated noise, or if Mitch came around a corner when I wasn't expecting him, or, worst of all, when my mother called my name.

The money my brother had set aside for the garage conversion ran out, of course, before the work was quite finished. The walls were up and the plumbing and electricity were in, but Mitch and I did all the drywall taping and mudding and then the sanding ourselves, working until well after midnight night after night, drinking wine, beer, vodka, the radio blaring. After that we primed and painted the walls, then scrubbed and scraped the cement floor, and primed and painted it. Then we lugged furniture, rugs, books, and put up curtains, all at top speed. My mother would wander in and out, admire the work, compliment us. This is going to be your little house, Mom, I'd tell her, brightly, guiltily, but it rolled right off her. I don't think it was merely a matter of faulty memory; she just plain didn't want to hear it. She'd wander away, then come back five minutes later.

"Tell me again," she'd say. "Why are you doing all this?"

When the night finally came to move her into the cottage, I felt as if I were putting her out on an ice floe. Stability and predictability, say the experts. This, including getting her out of her house in Connecticut, was move number four in seven months.

But Mitch and I were exultant. We crouched behind the car in the dark and watched her moving around inside the cottage. She's in! We did it! Our new era begins! I had laid out everything she'd need for breakfast, shown it all to her: oatmeal, honey, tea, butter, bread, eggs, bacon, bananas, all utensils, milk and orange juice in the refrigerator. She had a hot plate, a sink, a toaster, a blender. Polly nested happily on the sofa. There were familiar pictures on the walls, fresh sheets on the bed. She could be near us, part of the family, but independent! The last six weeks had been intolerably intimate, with no apartment to send her to, *nowhere* to send her to, but now, at last, she was in her new home, autonomous but not alone.

Early the next morning, I woke to cupboards banging. I flew out of bed and down the hall to the kitchen. She was in her nightgown, barefoot, bewildered. She was looking for something to eat.

When she had her apartment in town, she was constrained somewhat by not being completely sure how to get to our house. No more! The front door to the new house burst open twenty, thirty, forty times a day, every day: My mother, searching for her basket (which she has always carried instead of a purse), asking if she was having dinner with us, showing us a grocery list, asking if there was vodka in the house, telling us she was going to take a nap, asking the name of the doctor she saw last time she was here, showing us a grocery list, searching for her basket, telling us she wished she knew when she was going to die, asking if there was vodka in the house, showing us a grocery list, asking if there was a hospital in the next town, telling us she was going to take a nap, asking the name of the doctor she saw last time she was here, asking if she was having dinner with us, telling us she wished she knew when she was going to die, asking if there was a hospital in the next town, asking if there was vodka in the house, searching for her basket.

You find yourself doing things like putting a sign out in the driveway, at your mother's behest, with big black boldface letters, reading: "DINNER PARTY TONIGHT CANCELED!" Why? Because she'd come into the house after waking up from her nap insisting that she'd invited

ten people to dinner, but that we had no food, and so we had to do something to head them off.

Arguing was useless.

"No one's coming for dinner, Mom. If they were, I'd know about it."

I finally got it through my recalcitrant head that it was much easier, much more expedient, to find a big piece of cardboard and a Magic
Marker, make a sign, and put it in the driveway, let her help set it up with
bricks and a folding chair. Then she could relax, and then she'd forget.
Then I could slip out later and remove the sign. Until the next time.

Sometimes, amazingly enough, we actually did round up sympathetic
people and have dinner parties. She'd rise to the occasion, have a good
time, talking, sometimes dancing, doing what she loves best—socializing.
I'd see her in an intimate conversation with someone, and my heart would
give a little surge of joy. When the guests were gone, she'd sigh. "Well,
that was certainly a strange evening. No one said hello to me. No one
acknowledged me or spoke one word to me. I just sat there by myself for
the entire party."

My heart would plummet, my voice would rise. In an instant, I was
the child wanting to make her mother happy, and I'd failed.

"What do you mean? How can you say that? People were all over
you. You were the life of the party. That's crazy."

She'd shrug, make a skeptical little noise out of the side of her mouth
just as she'd done as long as I'd known her, and gaze away from me, forlorn
and pathetic.

September 1999: I'm sitting at the computer in my "study," a room in a
far corner of the house jammed with clothes, papers, books, unpaid bills.
A tap-tap on the door nearly sends me out of my skin. The floorboards do
not creak. They give no warning at all.

"El-Belle?" Her pet name for me. One of the sweetest sounds in the
world once. Now I leap as if someone had fired a gun in the hall.

"I'm right here," I say, summoning a pleasant tone.

"Listen, dear. I have a problem." She comes in and shuts the door, leans back against it, smoking a cigarette. She looks and sounds so absolutely normal. "Some woman came and borrowed all my letters from home and hasn't brought them back."

I close my eyes and gather myself before I answer.

"No one took your letters, Mom. They're all out there in your cottage."

"No. A woman came and took them."

"Now, why would someone do a thing like that?"

"She visited me, and I showed her the letters, and she said she'd like to take them and read them."

"Mom, if someone had come here I'd know about it. I seriously doubt there was any woman who took your letters."

"No, there was a woman."

"What was her name? What did she look like?" Here I go again. Arguing with a memory-damaged person, without a doubt one of the meanest, stupidest things you can do.

"Her name starts with a *C*. It's an odd name. That's why I can't remember it. 'C-r-e-e' something or other."

"You can't remember it because she doesn't exist." I despise the churlish, overbearing tone of my voice. My mother defends herself bravely.

"She came here when you were gone. She wanted to interview me for the newspaper. She wanted to know about where I came from, so I gave her the letters."

"Mom, if someone were going to interview you I'd sure as hell know about it."

"Well, she took them."

"No, she didn't."

"Yes, she did."

"She doesn't exist." I feel cruel. It's a powerful compulsion. I try to get a grip. "They're here. You've misplaced them. I'll help you look for them later. I think there's just been a misunderstanding."

"Well," she says, my conciliatory words apparently helping her save some face, "we'll see if you can find them. I can't. I've looked everywhere."

"I'll find them."

"They were in a big manila envelope."

"I'm sure I can find them."

This is maybe the fifteenth time we've had this conversation, a couple of times already that day, and it's my fault, because I haven't done what I know I should, what Mitch has told me I must do: Gather up a bunch of her unanswered letters from home (there are dozens and dozens of them), put them in a big manila envelope, and tell her they've been returned. Breathe life into the imaginary woman, too, if I must. Describe her hair and clothing. You learn that this is what you have to do. Truth is sometimes worse than useless.

On that first morning when she came into the house looking for food, I gently steered her back out to the cottage and showed her all her breakfast stuff. You should have your breakfast out here, Mom, I'd say. It's easier. Then dinner with us tonight, just like every night! It worked for a while, maybe a month or two. Sometimes she didn't emerge until eleven or so. A few precious hours for me to try to work, though of course I felt guilty every millisecond. But by then, guilt was my familiar old pal, a big heavy hairy arm draped around my shoulders twenty-four hours a day, and I'd learned to live with it.

We encouraged her to make her lunch out in the cottage too. It was a simple meal, the same one she'd made every day by rote for years. I always stocked her little kitchen with the necessary ingredients. That worked for a while, too. But soon I was fixing lunch for her, because she was forgetting even this routine, making weird disturbing blunders like trying to boil water in the cat dish or make oatmeal in the ashtray, putting the ingredients for spinach soup in her electric teapot instead of her blender and scorching the whole mess. Then she began to creep in at breakfast. Often she couldn't remember if she'd eaten or not, though I still faithfully laid out her food and utensils every night. I'd have to go out and look.

Sometimes she hadn't eaten, so I'd make her breakfast. And so it went, until I was cooking for her three times a day. I'd pretty much petered out on the brain nutrients and vitamins by then. They were expensive, made no difference at all, and it was one more disheartening routine. I did keep up with the antidepressants, but I might as well have thrown crumpled balls of tissue paper into a furnace.

She spent less and less time in her cottage. She lay on the window seat in our house, sometimes complaining about her stomach and asking about doctors all day. She didn't cry often when I was a child. Now she'd cry three or four times an hour, suddenly and with no warning. God, the perversity of her disease. Everything that made her a whole person was going or gone, but the memory of Mike and his death grew steadily sharper and newer every day.

"Why did Mike have to die?" she'd sob. "When I think of all the bastards who deserve to die." Then it would pass as abruptly as it began, a little tropical squall, and in the next moment she might even whistle an old Frank Sinatra tune. I, helpless, was jerked this way and that by every rise, fall, zig and zag of her emotions.

I was the nucleus of her universe. If I went down the hall and shut the door to get dressed, she'd forget where I was, get anxious, come looking for me, call my name through the door. If I went and locked myself into the bathroom, she'd go outside, circle around, and tap-tap-tap on the window. Her need for me and her vigilance wore me down, down. I could scarcely work, hardly read a magazine article all the way through, let alone a book, and my exercise routine was in shambles. Mitch's demeanor grew daily more grim, and I could scarcely blame him. Most men would have walked long ago. We drank, had horrible fights, lost sleep. I ran myself ragged trying to keep my mother away from him at the same time that I struggled to protect her from the knowledge that she had become—God have mercy on my soul for even forming the thought—old and in the way. I popped Valium day and night. Beautiful pharmaceutical; it unplugged my terror for a while so that I could function just a little. I think I might have keeled over dead without it.

She had an insurance policy that was supposed to cover long-term health care. It was useless, we discovered, for assisted living. It would only pay for a full-care nursing home, but it looked as if it also might pay for certified nursing assistants to come to the house and provide "companionship." We decided to try it. We could no longer afford Allen, her caregiver from the year before, and we'd already tried the local adult activities program, but they had tossed her out after a few days for being "uncooperative."

. . .

November 1999: The first CNA they sent was about eighteen but a tough little cookie. My mother was polite when we introduced the girl to her. Oh, she's really nice, the girl said about my mother. I left them alone together in the cottage. I went into the house and sat down at my computer. Twenty or thirty minutes went by when I was levitated from my chair by a screech of rage: "Leave me ALONE!"

So we tried having the girl take my mother out. Take her anywhere, we said—for rides, to the beach, the movies. She likes to get out. She likes action. She's always complaining that she's stuck here and never goes anywhere. So off they went, my mother with a shopping list, this time one I myself had contrived, and a few dollars in her pocket. Don't let her buy booze, we warned the girl.

An hour later the phone rang. My mother, demanding that we come pick her up, that she'd been abducted, that she had no idea where she was. I reassured her, told her all was well, that we knew where she was. Maybe an hour or two later, the exhausted girl brought her back. After she'd gone, my mother told a wild tale about being dumped in the middle of nowhere and having to hitchhike back to the house.

We gave up the experiment after a couple of weeks. It was much less harrowing to just keep her at home. She was back on the window seat, or shuffling back and forth between the house and the cottage, all day, every day, weeping, little flurries of sobs erupting out of nowhere, asking about stomach medicines and doctors, complaining that she was stuck here and never went anywhere.

February 2000: It's not even dark yet and I'm drunk. Earlier on this day, Mitch and I rode up to the assisted-living place where we left my mother last night. Our beat-up, old, ugly brown Toyota was completely covered with pink petals from the flowering plum tree it was parked under. The car looked as if it had participated in some sort of ceremony, something Japanese having to do with spring. Something festive and whimsical.

The day before had been one of lies and subterfuge. We had laid out our battle plan in advance: Mitch would take my mother out for three hours or so—shopping, errands. The instant they left, I sprang into action.

I dragged a big suitcase from under the bed, went out to her cottage, plundered her drawers and closet. Made instant selections: these pants, and these, and these, clean and presentable; these pants, and these, spotted, frayed, pathetic-looking. The good stuff into the suitcase, the sad stuff into a pile. Same with sweaters, shirts, underwear, shoes. The freight of sentiment at the sight of certain articles of clothing threatened to overwhelm me: a frayed cuff on one of her sweaters, artfully rolled to conceal the hole; a shirt she loved and wore for years, now stained and grubby. All signs of her slippage and my failure. She was, and still is, a snappy dresser. Even depressed and demented, she always puts together a jaunty outfit every morning.

I surprise myself with my fortitude. I make my selections, click the suitcase shut, stuff the worn dirty things in a box. I'll wash some, throw some out.

Then it's a sweep through the bathroom. Here's where I waver and slug down a shot of vodka. There's a Japanese word, *kawaisoo,* which, roughly translated, means "the pity of things." Here are prime examples: her lipstick, tweezers, toothpaste, hairspray, little bottles of makeup, combs, hairbrushes. The bathroom has been a source of unhappiness for me all along. We never quite finished it when we did the conversion, so desperate were we to move her out of the house and into the cottage, pressed for money and time and starved for privacy. When we painted the floor we were in a big hurry, and never got around to the corners and edges. We didn't put up trim, and there's a curtain instead of a door. Stray pieces of rug were nailed to the floor. The rug is now grungy, the unpainted corners of the floor dusty and fuzzy. I get out of there as fast as I can.

I grab the handsome African blanket from her bed, which she always neatly makes, every morning. She'd made it that morning, not knowing she would not be sleeping in it that night or probably ever again.

But I do it. Grab her folding chaise, her small Oriental rug, a tape player with a big-band tape in it, a TV table, and toss it all in the car. I go back into the cottage and pause in front of the photos she's put up on the wall: my brother and me as children and adults, old friends, and Mike, Mike, Mike. No pictures for now, I decide. Especially no pictures of Mike.

Mike, I ask one photo of him, the profile shot where he's outdoors wearing his tam-o'-shanter and looking very glamorous indeed, though he was a completely unpretentious guy, am I doing the right thing? I'm doing what the psychiatrist I took my mother to for a while advised her to do. Even though you're an atheist, the psychiatrist had said, and you have no belief that Mike is waiting for you in the hereafter or watching over you or any of that, you still have an image of him in your mind. And you can consult that image. You can ask it what Mike would say or do in a certain situation. And in that way you are communing with him. I remember thinking: Damn! That's a useful piece of advice. It was lost on my mother, but it wasn't lost on me. The image of Mike in my head, the wise, compassionate person I remember, said, Yes, you're doing the right thing.

At least, I think that's what the image said.

She'd been in the cottage for only about eight months, and we were throwing in the towel. The cozy haven we tried to make turned gradually and sadly into a prison cell. That's how she saw it. Squalor and clutter took over. Not horrifying; nothing to call the elder abuse hotline about, but not the level of dignity she deserved. Her housekeeping abilities slipped inch by inch, and so the job of keeping the place decent fell by increments to me, along with the cooking, and I was doing an inadequate job. I was also doing an inadequate job of keeping her hair, clothes, and body clean. If I didn't lead her to the sink and wash her hair for her, it didn't get done. And I didn't do it often enough. What I had feared for a long time was beginning to happen: That I'd get so burned out I'd neglect her.

A senile person with dirty hair is a tragedy. It embarrassed me, aroused pity, sorrow, and contempt in me, and I loathed those feelings and myself for feeling them. She has really nice hair, and when it's fresh and fluffy everything about her seems improved. So first I'd clean out her sink, full of stinky cat food cans, wet cigarette butts, crusty forks, and greasy frying pans. Then I'd announce that it was time to wash her hair.

And she'd bend over the sink while I sprayed her head. It made me sad to see the vulnerable nape of her neck. Then I'd fill my hand with shampoo and rub it into her hair. I knew she liked the touching and attention, but I found it disturbing to feel the contours of her skull. It brought unpleasantly vivid images to my morbidly imaginative mind. I'd think of her wasting brain just a centimeter or so from my fingers.

And when I made her take a bath, the sight of her naked body was tragic and disturbing to me, too. Although her muscles were atrophied, I could still see, in the line of her legs and the curve of her waist, the remnants of her beauty—the body Mike had loved. One night, months and months before we'd moved out of the old house and she was still living in her apartment a block away, she'd been undressing, and was standing there in her sweater and underpants, and I'd seen the gentle curve of her belly, and when I got home that night after putting her to bed I lay on the floor and wept helplessly for an hour. No one loves her anymore, I thought. No one in the whole world. Only me. I'm it.

The big picture is dreadful, but in the end it's the little stuff that finally makes you crack, voids all your grand plans and noble intentions. The senile person's world is a shrunken, fretful place, but it's all the person has, and so the vexingly trivial (to us) things in it are worried and worried like an old dog chew, and if the person is someone you really love, like your mother, for instance, then you're sucked right in there with her.

And when I say little stuff, I mean little. There was a routine we went through every day: She'd pick up, say, a rubber band or maybe a paperclip from the floor and ask: "Where does this go?" As soon as I'd shown her what to do with the rubber band or the paperclip, she'd find a plastic fork or a paper bag. "Where does this go?" Then a broken comb, or a piece of string, a bottle cap, a cork, an empty can, a pencil, until I wanted to shriek.

In the old days, when I was in trouble or needed help, I'd pick up the phone and call my mother. Every once in a while, I still get that crazy impulse: the Connecticut area code, the familiar little tune her number played on the touch-tone, her voice. Of course, I can't. I grieve for her exactly as if she'd died. She's gone, I've lost her, but I'm still responsible for her living, breathing body and the ghosts in her head.

You can't live with it. Take it from me, don't try. It will twist your love around and make you ill. Consider this a warning. You can't do it (unless

maybe you're grotesquely wealthy, though even then I wouldn't advise it).
I wish someone had warned me. Talk about stress—now, there's a word I
once tossed around casually without the remotest grasp of its true meaning. God knows what's going on in my own brain and arteries. I think I
can say without too much exaggeration that for now, at least by my own
standards, I'm an alcoholic and a drug addict. My wires and fuses are fried,
like someone hit by lightning three or four times. I'm inflicting the same
kind of harm on myself that my mother inflicted on herself after Mike's
death, maybe worse. I know it, but I do it anyway.

Mitch and I, pale and blinking like prisoners of war when the gates
are opened, sift through the rubble and assess the damage. Mitch's performance was nothing short of heroic, and he's assured me that he knows I
would have done the same thing if it had been his mother, but I can't help
it—I feel as if I sabotaged his life.

And it's impossible not to feel that I hastened my mother's decline
with my ham-handed attempt to save her. It doesn't matter what people
say, how much they try to reassure me. I failed her, and I know it. When
we started I wanted to restore her memory. Now I hope she'll forget—
Mike, Connecticut, everything. I still have nasty dreams—not real nightmares, but bleak little dreary desolate sepia-toned dreams, always at dawn,
when I wake as rudely as if someone had grabbed me by the hair, full of
dread and urgency. I've crossed into new territory from which there's no
turning back. My mother was essential to me in ways I didn't even know
about before. My fantastic fortune at having such a mother always con-
ferred a feeling of exemption. That's the only word that comes close. I felt
anointed, as if nothing really bad could ever touch me. That's gone now.
And my lens on the world has darkened a shade or two. A beautiful sunny
day and flowers blooming? I look at them and think, So what?

My mother will be on my mind every day for the rest of my life. I
understand now why people drink whiskey while they're still in their
bathrobes. And I also understand just how flimsy is the infrastructure of
cognizance, where our reason, memories, and identity lie. It's everything,
but it's a delicate and finicky synaptic soufflé. Once it falls, nothing will
make it rise again.

I'm also sick of hearing myself whine. I'm aware that I'm singing the white middle-class blues here. I could be in a mass grave in Bosnia. I could be on death row in Texas. I'm sure someone living in a tin shack in Haiti would really feel sorry for me. My share of good luck in this dangerous world is repugnantly disproportionate. I know that for a fact, but I still can't help it—we feel what we feel, and it feels as if my life's been punctured and time is hissing out wildly like escaping air.

March 2000: I feel like one of those guys on a doomed Antarctic expedition, the last one alive, writing in his diary right up to the bitter end. Maybe somebody will find this alongside my frozen corpse.

My mother's been in the assisted living place for a little over three weeks. The day after we took her there, she cried and begged to come home. The next few days were not so bad. I escorted her in to dinner on one of those nights and sat her down with the other old ladies at her table. They smiled and greeted her. I allowed myself a scrap of hope. People! Company! Attention! They all said it might be rocky at first, but that she'd adjust.

A day or so later, a fax from Sue, the head of the place: Your mother has been seriously agitated. We've put her on medication. Fine, I think, fighting back the alarm. Whatever it takes. Maybe that'll do it.

Next day, I go to visit. She's got her hat and coat on, and she's packed her clothes and toiletries into plastic bags and pillowcases. I want to come and try living with you, she says. She has no memory at all of the past seventeen months. I unpack her stuff while she cries and begs. Why can't I live with you? I'm all alone here, she says. All alone.

Calls at night: Announces she'll be checking out and going back to Connecticut to live with Joan Talbridge. The newspapers, she says, have reported that she's moving to California, but she's not. She's decided against it.

The next few days are a little better. A whole day goes by without any word from either her or the staff. My dreams and my sleep improve a little. I call her one afternoon, and Sue answers the phone in my mother's room. She's a little overmedicated, Sue says. I'm staying with her so she doesn't hurt herself. Whatever you need to do, I tell her, my heart flop-flipping like a netted fish, tacitly letting her know I'm not the litigious sort. Later, my answering machine flashing and flashing and flashing: Ten messages from my mother. *I'm all alone. I came all the way out here to visit you, and I'm stuck alone in this place. Oh, El-Belle! Where are you? Please, please call me.*

Next time I see my mother, she's quite good. Calm, lucid, more or less coherent.

Then, whammo! A call from Sue. Your mother attacked the night person on duty so that he (!) had to go hide behind a door. Was smoking in her room. Was out on her deck, banging on the railing, screaming ELLIE! ELLIE! ELLIE! Waking up everyone. Her medication adjusted again.

A few more days when things seem to be improving. Then, one morning while I'm visiting, Sue takes me aside, says she needs to talk business.

Your mother, she tells me, is the most high-maintenance person here (read: biggest pain in the ass). If she's going to stay, you're going to have to hire private-duty help, or come and fill in yourself. She's wearing out the staff.

And here's the part that I kind of knew was coming, that maybe I've known was coming all my life: she's frightening some of the other residents.

I'll sign off now. I've eaten the last of the sled dogs, and the wind is howling so that my lantern's flickering and the walls of the tent are about to blow down. I'm running out of lamp oil anyway. I'll just roll up in my sleeping bag and wait for morning, if it comes. I'll consult the image of my mother when she was in her prime. Mom, am I doing the right thing? What would *you* do?

I'm still waiting for the answer.

mourning in altaic

ED BOK LEE

There is a Korean proverb: *The best time to start is when you think it's too late.*

I never believed it.

My sister and mother took turns caring for my father after his esophagus was surgically removed. By the time I finally arrived in Florida, he was almost halfway through his chemo treatments, and could barely whisper. My mother and sister had earlier understood and agreed that my presence during the most crucial stages would likely only stress my father out. As far as he was concerned, I was unemployed: I split part-time shifts during the week at a homeless shelter and a package delivery warehouse in Minneapolis. On weekends I bartended in a Chinese restaurant.

Disappointing my father was nothing new. After high school, I left our North Dakota home and drifted, severely depressed, for nearly two years through Canada, the Pacific Northwest, California, Mexico, and throughout the South, taking mostly restaurant and temp labor work as needed. Only while physically moving to a new, unknown environment was there any kind of relief. I was almost always high. When it was warm enough out, I slept in the rear of my fold-down hatchback, and I regularly smuggled out a few days' worth of buffet chain food in an old gym bag. Something was deeply wrong, and my father never forgave me for it. By the end of the 1990s I'd tried to make a home in nine different cities. I eventually attended college but studied literature instead of pre-med, as my father had always hoped. Before his diagnosis of stage three cancer, I'd only seen him a handful of times over the course of several years, and on the occasions we did speak on the phone, it usually ended with his demand to know when I was going to start my life.

For all these reasons, when I finally did visit my dying father, I hung back to prevent any possible conflict.

While in Florida, I remember frequent swims in the gated compound's pool and catching up on reading in various cafés and used bookstores in and around Fort Myers. Anything to avoid my father's weakened state, which seemed only to magnify his disappointment in my presence. In his best moments, he seemed frustrated that he couldn't lecture me properly. In his worst, I'd have subjected myself to anything if only the intonations of pain emanating from his room could sound human again.

On the fourth day of my visit, my sister chastised me by the pool. "Why don't you go sit with him, maybe offer to take a walk together?" But I was too wounded by his accusation the night before at dinner, rendered in a crushing whisper, that I was a family embarrassment. A cold worm had slowly worked its way up my spine and entered my brain at his reminder that my "screenwriting" career clearly wasn't happening. And, for dessert, his favorite refrain: "Life is not a hobby."

Most days I slept until noon, taking full advantage of the recuperative silence of my father's rented condo. In the afternoons, I worked poolside on a play I was writing about a foreign military occupation of America. The Florida atmosphere, surreally appealing, inspired me with its tiny lizards leaping away from my bare feet in the grass; the languid humidity, which seemed somehow to make every character's essence linger more palpably on the page; the hydralike banyan trees whenever you suddenly looked up, certain that someone was staring.

I took a solo day trip to Hemingway's house in the Keys, with its many generations of eerie, inbred cats crawling everywhere, and finished writing a scene on a stone bench in the Old Man's garden. The climax I finished the next day in Sarasota, after touring the Ringling Circus Museum. It felt blasphemous that my writing was going so well while my family was suffering so. But I never once wanted to stop.

At night, I'd smoke on a lawn chair out by the compound's man-made lake, swim in the pool, or revise the day's writings at a tin-roofed, jerry-built bar nearby. Sometimes, if the writing was going too well to believe, I'd drink a couple of extra beers to calm myself and wander off to a movie.

There was a cute Latina with black, sugar-sweet eyes who worked at a sunglass-and-hair-extension cart at the mall; usually she'd be reading a novel to kill time. I'd slowly pass her shiny brown legs on my way to the cinema. One night I bought a pair of smudged sunglasses that she cleaned meticulously with a little cloth. It turned out she was taking a world literature class at a local community college; the book she was halfway through was *Crime and Punishment*. She was sunny like you hear of Southern girls, and I found my Northern ass circling back with a gift before her shift ended—*Lady with Lapdog and Other Stories* by Chekhov—from the mall's bookstore.

"He was a doctor," I told her. She said she thought she'd heard of *The Cherry Orchard*.

I mentioned my father's surgery and chemo, and, after ringing up a giggly teenage couple, she offered to show me around town sometime.

That Saturday we went to a club with her two hottie friends, one Vietnamese and one blonde, who, by their matching makeup and tans, similar voices, affects, and miniskirts, might as well have been twins from alternate universes. Afterward, without her friends, drunk and chain-smoking menthols on a park picnic table, she started tearing up over her own father's leukemia, how she and her mother recently learned that he'd had a second family in Puerto Rico her whole life. "And then the bitch tells me she never even married him, like legally!" Later, overlooking a dark ocean under a navy blue sky, we made out in my father's Honda. But she kept alternating between tearing up, apologizing, and half mounting me over the gearshift. Finally, two days later, she admitted over the phone that she was engaged to a guy her eight-year-old son called Dad. We made a date to meet at Starbucks, but she never showed.

My existence in Florida—there with my family, but not really there—felt strangely amphibian. I must have spent as much of my stay submerged underwater as I did wandering aimlessly, sun-drunk on land. Life seemed to be slowing and heightening, as if headed for a collision, but somehow at the pool, slipping underwater whenever difficult thoughts came, the impending blow seemed less inevitable.

In the compound's pool one night, vapors rising off the heated, sapphire blue water lit from below, it struck me how sad it would be if Fort Myers, where my father had no connection to anything, were to be his final resting place. He had moved to Florida several months before his diagnosis. For two years before that, he'd been living in Arizona and Texas, trying to shake the allergies that had tortured his senses for years. The plan had been that when he found a place where he could finally feel relief, my mother would retire from her job in North Dakota and move there. He'd been testing out Florida when the diagnosis of esophageal cancer came.

I brought the issue up with my mother and sister one evening over dinner while my father lay in bed recuperating from a chemo treatment. It seemed important to me—where his remains would *remain* after he'd passed on.

"Has he ever mentioned Korea, or North Dakota?" I asked.

Neither of them knew his wishes on this matter, nor seemed to care. Maybe I pushed too hard.

"We need to be positive." My sister finally spoke up, annoyed.

"Someone's got to think of these things," I protested.

Later that night, while my sister sat with my father, rubbing his legs, my mother and I spoke further on the matter. We spoke in Korean. In her native tongue my mother sounds happier, more girlish and carefree; her sense of humor flows freely into her personality. English deepens her voice's register, hardening and cooling the tone. English makes her sound more businesslike. In Korean, she's more likely to encourage.

But not always.

"He doesn't want to think about those things," she said. We were on the sofa together waiting for a Korean video to rewind to the beginning. If my escape during this time was writing, then these melodramatic miniseries from Seoul were hers. Sometimes she'd watch one after another until dawn. *"We should respect his wishes."*

From my father's bedroom, I could hear my sister's voice, higher than usual, as if speaking to a small child.

"Shouldn't we know, just in case?" I replied in Korean.

"I suppose."

"Do you want me to ask him?"

My mother thought about this. "Do what you want," she said in English.

The Korean soap opera's sappy opening melody drew my sister out, her finger over her lips.

Back in Minneapolis, I received updates over the next several weeks from my sister and mother on his condition. The cancer eventually returned, and so he was to begin another round of chemotherapy. I offered a couple of times to come back out and help, but the decision was left to me and, in the end, something always came up to delay a second trip. I did speak with my father on the phone a few times during that period, always in English.

My father's Korean was very different from my mother's. More curt, the language he intuitively reverted to when angry. I'd never been able to converse in Korean with him. I'd only attended kindergarten in Korea, never learning to read or write the language very well. When we moved to America—settling in the Midwest via California—it didn't take long for my sister and me to become fully committed to English. Later, when I was older and relearning Korean in college, on those rare occasions I'd try to speak my father's native tongue with him, he'd unfailingly reply in English, with neither malice nor sensitivity toward my efforts. He did this even after I returned from studying and working for a year in Korea in my early twenties; even after I'd worked diligently to relocate and strengthen the subtler, forgotten muscles in my tongue; even as I began writing letters to my mother solely in Korean—any attempt to communicate with my father in the language would always end in the same rutted topics, in the same rigid tones: my future, gainful employment, the need to settle down.

And yet I longed to speak Korean with him more now than ever—to access some part in him that, as had occurred in my mother, might help foster a different kind of relationship than the one we'd always had in America, in English.

Over the next couple of months, while his body struggled to repair itself, I made a point to call him regularly. On the phone, he seemed more preoccupied than usual. Even his typical, probing questions about my life in Minneapolis began to fade into vague indifference.

I assumed it was the cancer, and that he was dying.

But at the very end of his chemo treatments, the cancer unexpectedly went into remission.

In spring, my mother left Florida for two weeks to sell their house in North Dakota and fully transition out of her job. It was decided they'd live out the rest of their days in sunny comfort. She also needed a much deserved break. My sister couldn't help, having just accepted a new job in public relations back in California.

"Why don't you come spend time with him," my mother urged on the phone. *"He's okay, but lonely. I'll be back soon."*

It's clear to me now that both my mother and sister were still experiencing the relieved afterglow of the remission. They had, in tandem, done good, hard, patient work—and it had paid off. They had, in a sense, saved my father's life. And my father, although scalpeled open from navel to throat, had fought back against the odds like a champ. According to my mother and sister's reports, he was making regular trips to the beach. He took long walks around the compound. A loner all his life, he now even had another retiree friend he'd pal around with, Harold, who lived in the same mostly Jewish- and Italian-American gated retirement community. My sister still loves to tell how every morning Harold would pull up in the driveway and, after a few spry rings of his bicycle bell, my father would go to the garage, climb on his own bike, and, together, the two old men would ride off into the sunrise.

A number of people I've spoken with about losing a family member have confided that they experienced unforeseeable, seemingly unrelated changes in their own individual lives around the time of the event. Beautiful and tragic things—meeting the love of their lives, a divorce, job loss, blooming of old passions, a windfall, a bankruptcy, a new child, sudden relief from long-term affliction. In the case of adult children, it's as if the dying parent, in a strange reversal of birth, were now being pushed slowly back through the fully grown child, whose life as a result begins to manifest some new, profound transformation to fill the void.

A couple of weeks before my father's remission, my sister got engaged to be married. In addition, she'd made a career change, from high tech PR to food and restaurant PR in San Francisco, the latter field her true passion. My mother was about to retire, pack up, and move to Florida, where she knew no one and would have to start a new life. For me, everything simply began to slow way down. A low-grade depression set in that winter, followed by something I'd only heard of before—writer's block. At first, this provided a weird kind of peace, like being shut in during a snowstorm, but by spring it had poisoned me with the worst parts of myself.

For a few months, in and after my first trip to Florida, my creativity had flared like a cobra entranced. But don't many animals bristle and fang when actually most afraid? The "inspired" invasion play I'd finished during my first trip to Fort Myers had gone on to appear in a new play festival at the Public Theater in New York. But despite the talents of Paul Giamatti in the lead, the play was emotionally pinched, narcissistic, bent more on a cold, dark destruction of its characters than any true exploration of violence within a lambent cosmos.

Around this time, I also lost two of my jobs in Minneapolis. At the bar, I'd fallen into the habit of requiring a half dozen shots each shift to shine a high gloss over my personality. Because I brought in all my drinking friends to the bar, the owner tolerated this—until I got caught one night secretly doling out top-shelf liquor to a few folks I didn't even really know or like. At the homeless shelter—the easiest job I've ever had, complete with free lunches and dinners—my scant duties included making sure clients were out of bed and had vacated the premises each day by 10:00 A.M. One morning, sluggish from a hangover, I decided it would be all right to take a quick nap in an empty bunk during rounds, only to be nudged awake hours later—anonymous under the covers—by the unsuspecting supervisor who'd been called in to fill my absence.

· · ·

I arrived in Fort Myers for a second time in April. My last visit had been in December. Now the once friendly sun and heat seemed to pummel my every sense. On the way up to my father's door, panting, sweat dripping down my face into the cigarette between my lips, I overheard some neighbors discussing a small gator that had taken up residence in the man-made lake at the heart of the compound. The way they were laughing about it, I couldn't help but pity the creature lurking somewhere just below the small lake's glistening surface—for having come to this artificial hole in the ground with all the natural wetlands in the state.

I hardly recognized my father. Stunned by the sunlight, he backed away from the front door. He was alarmingly thin and swayed a little as I awkwardly reached to hug him, mostly to be sure he wouldn't actually fold in on himself. I'd been told he was walking more than a mile every day, but now saw that couldn't possibly be the case. I attributed the accelerated aging to the toll the surgery and chemotherapy had taken on his already weak frame.

"How long have things been like this?" I asked, looking around. All the curtains were drawn. A lifelong hunter, his three most-prized elk and buck racks peered ominously down from their mounts on a darkened wall.

"I don't know."

"Does Mom know?"

"Don't bother her. She'll be back. Nothing she can do."

That first night I searched the kitchen cabinets only to find several cans of Swanson's unsalted chicken broth. He'd thrown out all the Tupperware containers of food that my mother had prepared and placed in the freezer.

"I could not eat it," he claimed. "Too tough after frozen."

"Is this thing even plugged in?"

"Too noisy," he said of the refrigerator. "Cannot rest."

Inside the warm dark refrigerator there was a soft stick of margarine, a box of baking soda, a smattering of slimy, brownish broccoli fronds in the crisper.

He looked frightened, shriveled, childish in his too loose pajamas.

Still, he went to his wallet and tried to give me money to go out and get a bite to eat.

"Arby's nearby."

"I'm fine." I pushed away the bill he tried to place in my pocket.

In the darkness of his bedroom, he explained that an alternately dull and sharp ache throbbed constantly from deep within his abdomen, where his stomach used to be.

Upon removing his cancerous esophagus, the doctors had surgically elongated his stomach and attached it to his throat as a makeshift replacement. Now, he complained, the painkillers prescribed to him only caused piercing pain, dizziness, and nausea.

Slowly, he reclined in bed—upset, distraught, and weak from hunger, yet afraid to eat. Even a single well-cooked pea, he claimed, caused wrenching convulsions. Still, he refused the possibility of morphine—to his mind, the kiss of death.

"You have to eat something," I said, helpless.

"Got to heal first," he whispered, on his back, his eyes tightly closed. He was rubbing a healing stone over his pajama top where, underneath the fabric, white barbed-wire-like scars traced a line from navel to throat. It was shocking to see him doing this. Months earlier, he would have scoffed at such a thing as "black magic."

"Where'd you get the stone?"

"Your sister gave it."

Outside, over the front door, an octagonal yellow bagua mirror now hung to deflect bad energy.

I drove to a nearby Super Wal-Mart that first night. Lost in the giant, Jack-and-the-Beanstalk-like kingdom of consumer products, I nearly gave the senior citizen store worker a heart attack when I finally spotted her to ask where the Asian food section was.

"Say what?"

"Oriental foods, where they at?"

I'd read that fermented soybean paste, doenjang, was among the most nourishing foods for a body; it helps regenerate damaged nerve endings. I snap-rationalized that what would save my father now would be forms of the native foods he'd grown up with in Korea. Comfort foods. Over the years in America, he'd been forced to give up his favorite dishes, one by one, due to health problems. He'd given up salt, soy sauce, and red meat for high blood pressure. Rice and sweets for diabetes. And, finally, the biggest hits—his beloved kimchi and morning coffee—for esophageal cancer. No wonder he was afraid to eat. What taste was there left that he loved?

Since coming to America, my mother had gradually acquiesced to work around his increasingly bland diet, which he adhered to with religious zealotry. I thought if I could just get some of these old, earthy flavors and nutrients back into him he'd surely stop withering.

The best food I could find in the Super Wal-Mart grocery was powdered Japanese miso soup packets and spinach. Garlic and zucchini. Low-sodium soy sauce and beef bones for broth. Good enough. Back at the apartment, I shaved the thinnest sliver from a clove of garlic to add to the concoction. One of the few stories I remembered from Korea was of the Tangun, mythic founder of the nation, born to a bear-woman who had survived on twenty cloves of garlic and a sack of mugwort in a dark cave five thousand years ago. Koreans to this day eat garlic in some form with nearly every meal. Surely there had to be something to all this. During the Asian bird flu epidemic, hadn't Koreans been the least affected?

My midnight preparations on a tray, I knocked and entered my father's room.

"I told you I cannot eat," he said.

His thick white hair, which had barely been affected by the chemo, looked maniacal. He shifted from obvious pain in bed.

"You have to eat something."

"Maybe later." His eyes remained closed the entire time, his brow pinched.

I set the tray down by his bed, hoping the familiar smells would stir his will, but he only ordered me to take it away.

"How about a spoonful?" I gave one last try.

"No."

In the days to follow he was finally willing—and able—to take small mouthfuls of various dishes I prepared. In the kitchen, I'd experimented like Edison and his ten thousand versions of lightbulb filament. Things my father could take slow spoonfuls of: Gerber's Turkey Rice and mashed carrots, watered down; matzo ball soup in a jar; fish soup with grated turnips.

There was a Korean grocery store in the Bonita Springs area. I loaded up there and tried numerous versions of doenjang broth and other soups, but he sniffed at those bowls with exaggerated faces of disgust.

Mostly he lay in bed, his eyes tightly closed.

Sometimes he rubbed his stone back and forth over his chest.

My sister called regularly during my stay. Usually, it was from work; her office tone never failed to make me feel like a client. I explained he was losing weight.

"What did the doctor say?"

"They did some more tests. We're going back tomorrow."

"He likes bananas."

I asked as delicately as I could if he'd mentioned to her what, when the time came, he wanted done with his body.

"I'm sure it's in his will," she said.

"Mom said it isn't."

"You know, he really needs positive energy around him right now."

"If he doesn't know, we should come up with a few suggestions."

"I can't talk about this here."

"I think he needs to decide," I said.

"Why?"

"He's afraid. Don't you think there'd be some kind of comfort in knowing?"

"Just call me tomorrow after the doctor's report."

On the drive to the clinic he kept poking at the radio's tuner, never satisfied with any station. One AM shock jock was railing on about North Korea's nuclear program. He listened for a while, then switched the radio off in disgust. He'd lost so much weight, the heavy, polarized lenses in his eyeglasses overwhelmed his face.

His doctor wasn't there for the appointment. No specific explanation was given as to why. Eventually, another partner at the clinic sat us down in a hallway cluttered with stainless steel carts, between waiting and examination rooms. The young physician explained, mostly looking at me, that by all reports my father should have been able to eat without significant pain. He had no idea why this wasn't the case. He could prescribe a different kind of pain reliever, but nothing else.

My father had always possessed the greatest respect for the doctors and pharmaceuticals he so heavily depended on to adjust to life in America. My mother claims he was rarely sick and never allergic to a thing in Korea. Growing up, I remember his dresser top looking like a miniature metropolis of orange plastic prescription bottles of all sizes for hypertension, diabetes, frequent colds and flu, and his constant, punishing allergies, not to mention an assortment of other transient ailments through the years. Though they'd never completely cured him, the medicines had always kept whatever illness he had at bay. The surgery and chemotherapy had likewise eventually done this for the cancer. But now, here, as nurses rushed past with vacant stares, my 112-pound father couldn't even look the doctor in the eye. I could tell he was annoyed, upset, and possibly even hurt because his regular doctor wasn't there. He'd already felt, for some reason, that his doctor hadn't taken enough care in performing his surgery. Earlier on, this indignation seemed to fuel in my father a disgruntled kind of passion to heal. But now, before this young, unknown doctor squatting in sneakers before us in our folding chairs, my father didn't even seem to be listening to the questions I was asking about the possibility of a home IV.

During those nights before my mother came, I would enter my father's bedroom and sit with him, though mostly in silence. When we did speak, it was about necessary things: bills, car maintenance, his checkbook. It disturbed him deeply not to be able to balance his bank account on his own.

To fill the days and late nights I watched a lot of TV, gorging myself on the images. I tried to write, but still struggled. My pen could slip across and around any number of topics, ideas, feelings, and could even still do a few tricks, but piercing the surface to speak the truth I craved was completely hopeless.

I remember a bad dream my father had in which a shadowy figure behind a snow blower entered his room. "Should not have eaten," he said, though he'd only had a few sips of beef broth for dinner. I pulled my chair up beside his bed. "Why don't you try visualizing?"

On her last visit, my sister had taught him how to imagine his insides healing.

"Doesn't work."

"What about meditating?"

"I don't know how."

I'd had a girlfriend who meditated twice a day to control her craving for drugs and other exhilarations, such as hurling objects across the room at me. Sometimes, to help work on my own issues, I'd meditate with her.

"Hold your fingers together like this." I reached over and shaped his thumbs and middle fingers so they touched as two individual circles.

I began a simple chant.

"What's that?" he asked.

"Pali."

He thought for a while. "I cannot do that."

When I let go of his hands, he grimaced.

"Maybe you could pray," I said. I knew from my mother that his father had been an old-school Confucian, his mother a Buddhist, but his older sister a devout Christian.

"I do," he said.

"To whom?"

I'd gotten used to rubbing his legs without his having to ask, the skin astonishingly loose against sharpest bone.

"I don't know," he whispered.

It wasn't only writing I struggled with during this time. My eyes often glazed over while reading the dozen or so books I'd brought, the voices all so far away, as if I didn't fully comprehend the English language. One night I searched the bookshelves for something to read in Korean and came upon the chokbo my mother had shown me when I'd turned sixteen. Four bound volumes of my particular Lee (Yi) clan genealogy. My paternal grandmother had given them to my aunt to give to my mother, to pass on to me when she deemed the time was right. In the chokbo, as my mother explained, my family's bloodline was recorded by birth date, hometown, education, titles, and significant accomplishments—seven centuries back to the Koryo Dynasty.

My Korean name appears as the last entry.

I recall my interest piquing when my mother explained that my older sister wouldn't be receiving any part of the chokbo. Although the names of wives and unmarried daughters were recorded in more recent centuries, the bloodline and tradition were continued paternally. My mother described how my grandfather naturally assumed my father's older brother would pass the chokbo on to his eldest son, but that that uncle had developed into something of a black sheep and drunkard, bearing only one boy out of wedlock, then died after the war under mysterious circumstances. My father, the only other male—the bright, younger son—had never shown much interest in the chokbo. She conjectured that this was in part due to the fact that he'd grown up during the brutal Japanese occupation of Korea (1910–45). As a schoolboy, one day he'd been assigned a Japanese name and grammar book to learn the new national tongue, utterly confused to find himself seated in a classroom beside his servants' children. "They destroyed so much Korean culture and tradition in one generation," my mother hissed. She went on about how the Japanese subjugated, brainwashed, and exploited every soul and natural resource they could in Korea, enslaving tens of thousands of girls into sexual submission for the Imperial Japanese Army, assassinating the beloved Korean emperor and his family, even redirecting streams and moving hills to disturb the land's natural flow of energy. "Everything twisted, screwed up," she said. "Then came the Russians and Americans and the Korean War falling down on everything else!"

At the time, it all made little sense to me, living in Fargo, North Dakota: the chokbo's strange vertical rows of black calligraphy; the rooty, medicinal scent of the yellowed pages, printed and bound in the Korean year 4291 (1958)—only a fraction of the many more master documents in my father's hometown Hall of Records in Choongchung province. My mother traced her finger over my ancestor's brush-stroked poem from A.D. 1366, and slowly recited it. But I couldn't understand it, or read any part of the chokbo. I could barely read English. No one I knew read for pleasure. To be caught with a book meant ridicule. North Fargo was very working-class. I fell into almost every drug there was and drank myself into oblivion regularly from age thirteen on. Anything to stay away from home and the parents whose strange accents, ways, and rules had only served to heighten my sense of alienation. By my freshman year, I'd been placed on juvenile probation twice. One night in my junior year, while my father had me pinned against the basement wall with a loaded 12-gauge shotgun, screaming in Korean that a third offense meant juvenile prison, I unleashed a drunken, slurry torrent of four-letter words back in English that stunned him long enough for me to stumble out to my car and drive off.

We lived together another year under the same roof, until I was seventeen, but neither of us ever really came back from that night.

Now, sitting with my father in the evenings, I thought of posing direct questions about the Japanese occupation, the war's toll on his family, its violence. He'd never mentioned these things to me, or the older brother he'd lost. Nothing of his relatives or friends.

But looking at the scars scissoring up to his throat and the strain on his brow to keep the constant pain at bay, the idea of probing now, after so many years, felt invasive. I remembered all the times he'd inquired about my life, and I'd only grunted the bare minimum in reply.

Then one evening, without warning, he spoke. It was one of those rare times, his insides at peace, when enough nutrients still flowed through his blood and brain to make him fully lucid.

I was looking through a sports magazine, taking in stats.

"Mom said you're writing a novel," he said, dry-mouthed, without opening his eyes. "Do you like it?"

"I like writing."

He lay silent for a while.

"Maybe if you grew up in Korea it could be easier," he finally said.

"What could be easier?"

"Everything."

He swallowed and began slowly moving the stone over his chest.

"Still, you should marry a Korean girl," he added.

Emboldened by this rare mood, or maybe sensing vulnerability opening between us, I asked him as gently as I could where he would want to be buried when the time came.

He opened his eyes, and thought about it, blinking at the ceiling.

"You guys decide," he finally said, closing his eyes again. "Maybe by water. I don't care."

He grimaced.

To change the subject, I asked what he thought about all day. The good things. Here. Now. With his eyes closed most of the time. I suppose I was still hoping to hear something about his childhood.

"What gives you some, any kind of relief?"

After a moment, a faint smile eased the strain on his forehead.

"You know, fishing," he said, without opening his eyes. The stone now lay motionless inside his fingers on his chest. "With you guys. So cute. All of us. Good things like that."

A few days later my mother arrived. I remember her shifting countenance when she first saw him—shock and sadness; how these emotions flickered and reared, then, just as quickly, submerged again. I'd trimmed his hair the day before. Smoothing down his luminous white mane in the sunlight with her two hands and a smile, she looked twice as young, a girl grooming her favorite doll.

I left them alone, but listened to my father's voice through the door—more plaintive with her now than ever with me. More frightened and childlike.

He told her about the problem he was having balancing his checkbook.

She asked him what he and I had been doing, of the trip to the clinic.

As I listened to their voices tenderly reconnecting, it suddenly oc-

curred to me—not only *how* they were speaking, but *what*. Not the Korean they'd used with one another my whole life. Instead, now my mother
would ask him questions in Korean, and he would answer in English. Or
she might start something in English, and a Korean reply would come.
But, more often, their sentences were jumbled—a strange, subtle dance
between languages and cultures; all unconscious to either of them. Or
maybe it was a kind of competition. Not between the two of them. But
between the people they'd become and who they once had been.

The genealogical classification of Korean remains uniquely uncertain.
Linguists continue to debate its origins—some scholars place it in the
Altaic language family, while others define it as a language isolate. Mor-
phologically, it possesses more similarities to Finnish than Chinese, despite
all geographical logic. In short, it is one of a very small number of world
languages that have no traceable lineage to a knowable past.

I left a few days later, planning to return when the time was right.

I didn't mention to my mother that I was taking the chokbo with me.
I knew that she'd meant for me to keep the books years and cities earlier.

I took some photographs of my father from a family album as well.

I've heard that it's perfectly natural to remember a dead loved one
once or even several times a day for the rest of your life. Yet many people
over time begin to feel indulgent for doing so. They begin to worry that
it means they're not letting go, moving on with their lives. Much needless
guilt and suppression can result. Ironically, at the same time, it's perfectly
normal, after only a few short years, to begin to forget exactly what the
loved one looked like at the end of life. You always remember the person's
essence and personality, the spirit. But the face and voice possessed at the
time of death begin to fade and blur into a lifetime of other memories of
the person—replaced, finally, in recollection, by a memory of the face in
the photograph you most often look at, the voice owned at that particular
moment.

It's a subtle, unconscious shift.

Like language. Culture. One period of history into the next.

I close my eyes and try to recall the first time he took me fishing.

My fingers slipping inside larger hands around one steadying rod.

This would be in Minnesota, possibly California, not likely North Dakota or Korea.

But I'm not sure anymore. Not even of the language we share.

It doesn't matter.

Soon evening will lead us home.

don't worry.
it's not an emergency.

SUSAN LEHMAN

My mother lived on sorbet, doughnuts, and cigarettes—four packs a day!—for twenty years. Also, except to eat sorbet and doughnuts and to get an ashtray in which to snuff out a cigarette, she pretty much didn't move. She was not in good shape to begin with, but still, it took decades before her weird suicidal regimen actually worked.

Long before she died last spring, I moved my mother into my apartment building. The idea was to set an example for my three young children. I wanted it to occur to them, when I was old and useless, that it might be a good idea to install *me* somewhere nearby and keep gentle watch over me.

Can you imagine how strange it would be to find your mother's couch on the sidewalk outside your New York apartment building? I don't know why the moving men left the couch and the other material remains of my mother's seventy-nine years in Toledo, Ohio, on the sidewalk when she came to live with us. But the sight of the couch—its absurd cotton flowers blooming over East Ninety-seventh Street in New York—was as dramatic (if less expected) as the spectacle of her protracted death.

It had, of course, occurred to me that having my mother on-site might present problems. Never in a million years, however, could I have imagined, when I saw the couch on the sidewalk that signaled my mother's arrival, how very gruesome these problems might be, or that they might involve armed police officers and large men with morphine. Nor could I have guessed how oddly rewarding the project of caring for someone who is nutty and sick might be for my three children, whom my mother lured upstairs with donuts, Tootsie Pops, and the promise of endless supplies of other sweets.

It started with a phone call.

"Don't worry. It's not an emergency." Obviously if you are in your right mind and a voice you don't recognize says something like this to you, you should hang up. *Right away.* Especially if the voice then says, "You're mother has had a little fall."

If the next thing you hear is that your mother, who is seventy-five and recently widowed, is about to be airlifted off a faraway island and deposited in a hospital *right around the corner* from your apartment—well, either you are in a Philip Roth novel or you are in real trouble.

I didn't hang up when a man called from the Teterboro Airport in New Jersey in the spring of 1999 to tell me about my mother's imminent arrival in a medevac plane. Instead I said, "Okay. I'll meet you in the emergency room." (I lived around the corner from New York's Mt. Sinai Hospital, formerly known, as I learned during the course of my mother's eight-month hospital stay, as The Jews Hospital.)

My mother had gone with a friend on vacation, the first she'd taken in twenty-two years. She'd lasted two nights before she crashed down on a bungalow floor, shattering her bone and providing the island's emergency medical personnel with useful occupation. The island doctor called to the scene apparently suggested amputation.

This would be a good place to describe my mother's voice. Really it wasn't so much a voice as a thunder. A *blast,* a word she herself often used, captures it best: loud and alive with grand, hyperbolic force.

Doctors say hearing is the last sense to go, that until the very end, a dying man hears—and, hopefully, finds comfort in—the softness of nearby voices. My mother's voice was not soft. I can't re-create its force, or even her exact remarks, though I know for certain that the words *amputate* and *bungalow doctor* boomed through the emergency room the afternoon my mother arrived, and I bet too that the muscular orderlies who rolled her in were surprised to find themselves laughing loudly and a lot in response to an old woman with a shattered leg, delivering a lively, ludicrous, over-the-top but somehow exactly on-point disquisition about island doctors who like to amputate.

There followed a series of long days full of rage and comedy, of doctors and nurses and orderlies and a constant screeching *crrkkkkzz frsssx* from the intercom on the wall in the room my mother shared with innumerable roommates—including one who screamed in the night, a woman dying, slowly, apparently agonizingly, and without the company of relatives or friends, of cancer—until at last my mother was released.

On that day, I took her downtown in a cab—a wonderful friend of my mother's offered her a spare room in her apartment while she recuperated. "Bye, Mom. Enjoy. I'll talk to you later today," I said and skipped out, enjoying the sense that each block between Washington Square and East Ninety-seventh Street represented a universe away from the hospital and that awful season of doctors and tests and bad smells.

Four seconds after I left, however, my mother fell down on her friend's bathroom floor, smashing her "good" hip (the right one), as well as her right leg, to bits; and so, before I even got back to Ninety-seventh Street, my mother was in an ambulance, on her way back to Mt. Sinai for another three months of groaning roommates, viral smells, and expensive flowers wilting next to uneaten trays of hospital "food."

By the time she was released from the hospital the second time, no one wanted to take any chances on excursions downtown or alternate recuperation venues: My mother was going home to Toledo.

She lived alone there, but we could hire someone to help. After the eight months at Mt. Sinai, I would not have been sorry if the doctors had decided to send my mother to Alaska. Or Neptune.

During the first few days after her return to Ohio, I developed a near phobic terror of ringing telephones. *Don't worry. It's not an emergency.* What if someone called to say that now?

I had a husband and two small children, a double stroller to push instead of a wheelchair at Mt. Sinai. Trust me. After what I'd been through with my mother, it was thrilling to go to the playground with the kids, to catch fireflies and eat ice cream cones and blow soap bubbles in the evenings while my mother was busy smoking, eating her donuts at a nice safe distance, six hundred miles away.

"Everything is hard," she complained on the phone. "I can't move. I never thought I'd end up like this." (Really? I thought. Did you imagine, after years of cigarettes and donuts and your refusal to move, you would end up on an Olympic soccer team?)

Children, as my kids were soon to show me, know the truth about most things. I soon realized that I could not live in terror of ringing phones, and also that my mother couldn't take care of herself—or climb stairs, for that matter, so she slept on a broken couch on the ground floor of her house. This is also where she sat all day—or more properly hung in a weird up-side-down way, for reasons connected with a back ailment of mysterious provenance—and watched television and raged at Republicans and doctors and smoked cigarettes. I also knew that this was not a terrible situation and that generally, if you can help it, it's better if your mother does not die alone on a broken couch in a room with gummy, nicotine-stained walls in a house in Toledo, Ohio. And I knew that, aside from me, there were no other plausible candidates for the job of taking care of my mother, and that having her in the building might make a good, useful impression on my children.

All of which is to say that what began with the *don't-worry-it's-not-an-emergency* phone call from Teterboro ended with my flying, in the spring of 2000, with my six-week-old baby, Max, bundled in a Snugli, to Toledo to pack up my mother's house and bring her and her broken couch with the crazy flowers to New York.

When I unpacked my mother's suitcase, I found giant bags of candy inside. My mother quickly turned her one-bedroom apartment into an infant vice den. Every day for the next six years, she lured Zack, Annie, and Max upstairs with fruit-flavored Mentos, Twizzlers, Tootsie Pops, doughnuts, and who knows what else. And, every day for the next six years, Zack, Annie, and Max got into the elevator and went happily upstairs to eat candy and doughnuts and watch TV and, for all I know, smoke cigarettes with my mother.

Did I mention that my mother had no teeth? And that as a result, her mouth flapped back and forth, like bird wings, over her face? Did I mention that my children called her Doodles?

They did. Her name was Doris. At some point, though, she must have suggested the boppier nickname, and it stuck.

"Doodles, put your teeth in!" I must have said this 412 times a day, during the first few months after she moved in. My mother kept hers—a clump of plastic nougats strung together on a gold wire—in a round, blue plastic box that was never, *ever* anywhere nearby and that required what, for her, was superhuman strength to retrieve. You may not know it, but chances are, you have strong views about people and teeth and chief among them is the idea that, unless you have just had a motorcycle accident or are George Washington, people should have them.

The flapping drove me nuts. Not just because it gave my mother the freakish, grotesque look of someone *very* far down on their luck, but because each back and forth jut of my mother's jaw signified her complete refusal to comply with the most minimal demand imposed on functioning participants of everyday life.

The remarkable thing about my mother and her teeth was not that, within six months of her arrival, her false bridge broke in half and she declared herself too weak to go to a dentist—thus putting an end to the entreaties, "Doodles, *please* put your teeth in"—but that neither the flapping nor the toothless gap made the slightest bit of difference to any one of my three children.

"Doodles!" five-year-old Zack would say and run to the elevator. "Bay!" (Meaning sorbet.)

"Polly Wolly Doodles!" Three-year-old Annie's face lit like a little sun in the middle of her music class one day. "It's a *song* about Doodles!"

"I'm going to upstairs. I'll be on eight," two-year-old Max would say, stamping his little feet when, in the midst of a tantrum, it occurred to him he could run away—without having to leave the building.

On eight. It was a phrase the kids used constantly during the years my mother lived upstairs. *On eight* meant on the eighth floor, at my mother's apartment. But it was also a state of mind.

On eight meant away from home, away from the jackhammer *blahblahblahblah* sound of parental voices. *On eight* meant a parallel world in which children had more power, by which I mean literal motor power, than the resident grown-up.

What did they do up there besides eat candy and watch TV? My mother never read to them. Not once. Too much physical activity. Nor did she ever play a game with any one of the three children. "I don't know how to play," said my mother—1932 Northwest Ohio spelling bee champ, Radcliffe graduate, and former assistant to Eleanor Roosevelt—when her four-year-old granddaughter asked her to play hangman.

Nothing said "state of eight" better than the scooter my mother bought in the spring of 2003, when it suddenly occurred to her it might be nice to go outside, to watch the kids play in the park, or just to be on the street, where, after two years in New York, her couch had, in fact, enjoyed more time than she had. So she bought a scooter, a bright red motorized wheelchair with a horn that made a cheerful *beep beeping* sound.

Beep beep beep, she honked when she rode the scooter through the lobby, Max on her lap, the day the medical-supply people came to show her how it worked.

Of course, my mother never rode the scooter again after that.

The kids, however, put it to immediate good use. In the image I have of this time, the kids whirl around my mother's apartment in a mad continuous loop, Zack at the scooter wheel, Max shrieking with laughter behind him, as they zip through the apartment—*beep, beep, beep*—crashing into walls, laughing their little heads off while my mother sits at the dining room table smoking a cigarette and explains to the visiting physical therapist that no, she cannot lift her right arm (or, for that matter, her left arm) above her head. "This is Maxi, the love of my life, and Zack, who used to be my friend," she'd tell the therapist when the boys pulled up at the table after completing a satisfying loop in which the children traded energy and life—in fact, *reason* to live—for endless sweets and endless love.

Things changed. Annie and Zack got older and went to school. My mother felt betrayed. "You abandoned me," she'd tell Zack and Annie when they got home from kindergarten and nursery school as if it were appropriate to give four- and six-year-olds the idea that going to school constituted abandonment. "Max is still my friend," she'd say, apparently also oblivious to the notion that it might not be wise to tell a three-year-old that an old woman's life depended on him. But the kids seemed as little bothered by my mother's warping remarks as they were that there was a hole in her face where most people had teeth. Max came home from music class on Valentine's Day with a clay sculpture heart that said "Max and Doodles forever" in gold glitter letters.

During her first two summers in New York, my mother came with us when we went to the Berkshires in August. By the second summer, the last she spent with us there, my mother had deteriorated so much so that the arrival at a beautiful carriage house high on a hill in a forest of pine and fir trees served as the occasion for high drama. The house was at the end of a rutted road. I couldn't drive my mother to the door. She couldn't walk up the hill. It was going to be hard to push a nearly three-hundred-pound woman in a wheelchair up a rutted road.

"Don't worry, Doodles. I'll push!" said Max, hopping out of the car, improbably offering to push a woman ten times his weight up a hill in a chair.

"Don't worry. I got you," he said, extending his little arm to pull her through the door after I had, at last, pushed her up the hill, Max in front of me holding tight to both the chair and the idea that *he* was doing the heavy lifting.

"I'm Dr. Zack. Here to see my grandmother," my oldest son told the receptionist in the lobby of Mt. Sinai, where Doodles, sick with pneumonia, went again in the fall of 2002.

"Okay, Dr. Zack. Go on up," said the receptionist. Zack, who no doubt would have rather whirled around the living room on eight than walk through a scary-smelling place full of sick old people, marched forth, plastic doctor kit in hand, as if it were assumed that when someone who is part of your life goes somewhere else, you take your kit and go *there*.

Doodles's hospital bed, which moved up and down, was a source of great amusement. "Look," said my mother, pressing a button and sailing upward on her bed. Zack took a turn, laughing as my mother went up and then down and then up again, high enough finally to send the IV pole attached to her arm smashing into a fluorescent light fixture. The fixture shattered into a thousand pieces all over the hospital bed and floor—which sent my mother's roommate into a loud, semihysterical remembrance of Kristallnacht. Orderlies rushed in with gloves and dustpans, and a stern nurse arrived to see what had happened. "I did it," my mother said. "I pushed the buttons." Zack, who may have assumed hospital visits were part of the order of things, apparently hadn't guessed his grandmother would take the bullet for him when he pressed too many buttons and glass rained down. "Thanks, Doods," he said when the nurse followed the orderlies out with dustpans full of glass.

Probably it was as much fun for the children to make hospital visits as it was for me to race upstairs and pick my mother up when she fell, which she did every now and then after she returned home. At 265 pounds of more or less dead weight, it was a job to get her off the floor. She was good at screaming things like "You're killing me!" "I can't. I can't. I can't move. I'll just stay here!" The officers who arrived once when I called 911 clearly suspected the large woman laughing on the floor—"I'll just stay here. Hahahahaha!"—might be drunk or loopy from drugs. Moments after they'd hoisted her up and put her back in her chair at the dining room table, Doodles lit a cigarette and offered the policemen drinks. "You need one after all that heavy lifting," she told them. *Hahahaha.*

Do you remember the blackout during the summer of 2002? All the power in New York City shut down. Doodles, who had announced herself too weak to be carried out of the building that summer and conveyed in a car to our rented house in the country, was alone when the lights went out. There was no way to tell her what was happening because her phone, which was cordless, didn't work.

"Let's save Doodles," said Zack, a mission that thankfully (by my lights) was aborted when New York EMT arrived to help. They carried my mother, who had trouble breathing without assistance from an electrically powered machine that shot nebulizing chemicals into her lungs, down eight flights of stairs and took her back to The Jews Hospital, which had become her home away from home.

If this had been a play, the blackout of 2002 would have been a good theatrical device, signaling that matters were beginning, at this point, to darken in the life of Doodles.

Neither Zack with his kit bag—or the doctors with theirs—could figure out precisely what was wrong. Batteries of tests were ordered. The results were inconclusive. Why couldn't this woman walk? The answer remained as mysterious as the ongoing riddle: Why couldn't this woman lift her arm or get on a scooter and ride outside for an ice cream with her grandchildren?

"She needs candy," the children decided, and arrived at the hospital with Tootsie Pops and clumps of chocolate fudge they got at a candy store around the corner.

We might all learn from children the interesting habit of accepting things as they are. As in: Why didn't Doodles move? "I don't know," said Zack. "She just can't."

Doodles, however, accepted exactly nothing, not the eminently reasonable suggestions to get up and try to walk with a physical therapist, or to try to eat something sort of healthy, or not to smoke cigarettes in the bathroom because it is against hospital rules—not to mention the law.

The ongoing failure to find a diagnosis, much less an effective treatment for whatever it was that ailed her, coupled with condescending remarks from orderlies and nurses, all of whom seemed overworked and underpaid and subject to unbearable abuse and desperate pleas from a steady stream of sick and dying patients, many of whom screamed pitiful things all night long like "Nurse, nurse, I'll make it worth your while, please please please help me . . ."—well, I'm afraid this did not bring out the best in my mother. Her mind was in full force; it was her bones, her exhausted lungs, and her considerable flesh that were rotting away. And she did not take well to being treated like a foolish child when she said understandable things like "Nurse, I'm having trouble breathing. When you get a chance, I need a nebulizer treatment."

"*Goddamn it*, I went to Harvard," she'd snap when the nurses, who addressed patients in sing-song voices usually reserved for children under the age of two, said things like "There, there. Be a big girl now. Nurse Sing-Song will be back soooon."

"Big girl needs candy!" said Annie, offering a big chunk of fudge wrapped in pink paper from the drugstore.

Step on a crack, you break your mother's back. The EMT guys who carried my mother home after her second-to-last hospital trip must have stepped on a crack. She arrived screaming in pain and couldn't move. The doctor who visited worried it was a fracture and administered morphine. Suddenly, Doodles had that faraway street junkie look and nodded when the kids showed up to welcome her home and sang "Deck the Halls" by her bed. "'Tis the season to be jolly, Fa la la la la, la la la la." Nod, nod, nod.

Despite the morphine, Doodles continued, as always, to understand the bottom line, essential facts of all matters. For example, when the EMT men arrived, two days after they brought her home, to carry her out again, this time to the Jewish Home and Hospital for the Aged, where it was suggested she might benefit from a rehab program, they took all kinds of precautions, beginning with a nice big morphine dose, to keep Doodles comfortable during what would be the interesting acrobatic feat of getting her out of bed without moving—or touching—her fractured back. Still, Doodles screamed. "OOOOCH! Agony! I'm in agony. AHHHRCHHH."

"But, Doodles," said my husband, who was there to help, "they're not touching you!!"

"I know," she said, "but they're *thinking* about it."

"Why does Doodles get a new house and we don't?" Annie said when I told her Doodles had moved to the Jewish Home and Hospital. The morphine addled her still fierce mind, but Doodles apparently appreciated the question when I relayed it to her   its charm and great goofiness—and smiled and laughed, weakly, in response.

The kids came to say good night an hour or two before Doodles died. Max, the little one who had stayed home and watched *Dora* and *Caillou* with Doodles and had not betrayed her by going to school, threw the first shovelful of dirt on the grave. A flutist from the Toledo Orchestra played Bach's "Jesu, Joy of Man's Desiring" while a rabbi said something or other in Hebrew, a nice comic note Doodles certainly would have enjoyed. The children suggested a piñata for the funeral, but instead put daisies, Doodles's favorite flower—"so cheerful," she'd said—on her grave.

It amazes me that, more than a year after her death, Annie and Max and Zack still cry so often, especially when they are going to sleep. They say things like "I wish I could tell Doodles I wrote a book about pilgrims in school." Or "You won't get me a computer? Doodles would have." Or simply: "I miss Doodles." This is often followed by tears and a statement that is the perfect articulation of loss: "I want everything to be like it always was."

Am I making pretty what was an awful spectacle of life-warping depressive illness, an unpleasant burden borne by children? Maybe. But my mother, with her vast unmoving helplessness, attendant rage, abiding humor and dependence, left my children with a sense of the sweetness—and the headache—involved in caring for someone else.

I think of three-year-old Max, standing at the bottom of the road in the Berkshires, offering to push my mother up a mountain in a chair, a perfect image of the way in which attending to a sick but loving nut-bar (*Here lies a nut*. Doodles asked that these words be inscribed on her grave) was for Max—and all of Doodles's grandchildren—a confidence-building enterprise that showed them how much *they* had to give.

Two weeks after she died, Zack went to eight to get a book he kept there and returned with a great big grin, his gob stuffed with something. "Zack," I said, "what's in your mouth? What's so funny?"

He smiled and said, crunching on something sweet-smelling and fruity, "The last of Doodles's candy!"

in the land of little girls

ANN HOOD

My daughter's blond hair has turned pink from blood.

"You can wash it tomorrow," a nurse tells me.

I nod, but I can't seem to stop playing with Grace's hair, smoothing it, rubbing the fine, pink strands between my fingers.

The nurse has me by the elbow now, urging me firmly away. "Tomorrow," she says again. "You'll see. That comes right out."

Ever since Grace arrived in the ICU almost twenty-four hours ago, nurses and doctors and social workers have been moving me away from her. And I have been shaking their firm grips off my arm, pushing past them, staying by my daughter's side. Grace is five years old. Until a few hours ago, we were told she wasn't going to live. But now they are talking about what lies ahead for her, and us, over the next few days. They are saying the word *tomorrow*. I let the nurse lead me to a chair across the room from Grace. Machines beep steadily. The ventilator gasps. I watch the rise and fall of my pink-haired daughter's chest, relieved and exhausted.

In the land of little girls, mothers do almost everything for them.

I still had to put Grace's socks on for her.

I made her breakfast every morning.

I shouted for her to stop at street corners when she raced ahead of me.

I cut her pizza and her pork chops and her cucumbers into bite-sized pieces.

I sat at the bathroom door while she took her bath.

I combed the snarls out of her hair, took her glasses off her each night, watched her make her slow, careful way down the steep steps of our two-hundred-year-old house.

On Tuesday, April 16, her brother Sam's ninth birthday, I took Grace to her ballet class in a church hall like I had every Tuesday for three years. The church is located on a street near Brown University, and parking is difficult. On this Tuesday, it was especially hard to find a space, and we circled the student-clogged streets over and over.

I had already considered having Grace skip her lesson that afternoon. That morning, she seemed lethargic. In fact, she had given Sam his birthday present from her bed. When I picked her up from kindergarten, she told me she'd had a long day. Back at home to get her ballet bag, I couldn't find a pair of clean tights. "I've got to have tights," she told me, and right then I thought: Keep her home this afternoon. I had to get Sam's birthday party ready. Unusually warm weather had given us the idea of having a cookout, and our kitchen was full of hamburgers and hot dogs, rolls and chips, as if it were a summer day.

But I found a pair of clean tights way in the back of Grace's drawer and raced back downstairs waving them triumphantly. I had to get the laundry done. Had to buy Sam's birthday cake at Ben & Jerry's, had to bake the artichoke dip he and Grace loved. And, circling the streets of our neighborhood, I had to find a parking space.

The one I finally found was several blocks away, so I took Grace's hand, and we ran to the church. Inside, I pulled off her new striped capri pants and her bright pink shirt and began the clumsy process of getting her into her leotard and tights. Grace held on to my shoulders, the tights twisted awkwardly, the leotard rolled. It was a weekly challenge, this rushed dressing followed by the climb up the stairs through all the other little girls dressed in pale ballet pink. On this Tuesday, I tried to pull Grace's hair into a ponytail. Only girls with long hair got that privilege, and Grace had been growing hers all year. But it still wasn't quite long enough.

"Maybe next week," I told her, foolishly believing that we would be here again next week, in this church near Brown University, struggling into leotard and tights like we had been every Tuesday for three years;

foolishly believing that one of these afternoons, I would gather Grace's pale blond hair in my hands, pull it away from her face, and magically, finally, it would fit into a ponytail.

Then I followed my daughter up those stairs and watched her skip into the large hall for class. Dust motes danced around her like fairy dust in the sunlight. The ballet teacher said, "Hello, Grace!" And the heavy wooden door closed on my last image of my daughter as a healthy five-year-old little girl.

That afternoon, after Grace went into ballet class, I ran down the stairs, out of the church, and onto Thayer Street, the main drag for Brown University. Past the store that sold incense and bangle bracelets, past Starbucks, past the Indian restaurant that sent the smell of curry and coconut into the warm spring air, past the stale popcorn smell of the Avon Cinema, past the Gap, the bookstore, the other bookstore, to Ben & Jerry's, where I picked up Sam's birthday cake and then ran, sweating, awkwardly holding the box with the cake sliding around inside it, all the way back down Thayer Street to the church.

We mothers all waited for our little girls in the hallway outside the room where the class was held. We sprawled on the scuffed wooden floor and lined the stairs leading up. When I turned the corner into the hallway, the other mothers all looked at me in a way that let me know something was wrong. But before I could ask them what had happened, the door swung open and the ballet teacher, Mary Paula, appeared.

"Good," she said, and motioned me inside.

Little girls in pink leotards were everywhere. But I couldn't find Grace's blond head in the swirl of pink. Mary Paula was walking away from the little girls, across the sprawling room, and I followed, confused, until I saw where she was headed. Under one of the enormous windows, stretched out on a stack of folding tables, lay Grace.

"She fell," Mary Paula was saying. "And she landed on her arm."

Her arm. It was broken. I could see that. I realized I was still holding Sam's birthday cake. I was remembering how far away I'd had to park. I was noticing how dull Grace's eyes looked, how still and quiet she lay.

"Grace?" I said.

She nodded.

"Are you all right?"

She nodded again.

"My car," I said to Mary Paula. "It's way down on Power Street."

"Go get it," Mary Paula said. "I'll bring her down and wait for you."

I ran. Out the door, holding Sam's birthday cake. A broken arm, I kept thinking. Not the worst thing that could happen to a little girl. So why did I feel so scared? There was so much to take care of that I just began doing those things: calling my husband, Lorne, to meet us at the ER. Calling my cousin to cancel the birthday party. Getting the car. Running back inside and scooping my daughter into my arms oh so carefully. All of those mothers' eyes on us. I said something to them, something about a broken arm. I buckled Grace's seatbelt. I stopped at home to put the birthday cake in the freezer and to get Grace's stuffed dog, Biff, and the book of Charles Addams cartoons that she loved.

Then I drove to the ER, glancing back at Grace in the rearview mirror the whole time. Thinking, *Something is wrong.*

That night, the last night Grace was ever at home again, after her arm was declared broken and we were sent home, we all ate birthday cake together. In a strange stroke of bad luck, Lorne's car was stolen while I was at the ER. We all laughed at Sam's exciting birthday: broken arms and stolen cars. Grace finally asked to go to bed, and Lorne carried her upstairs. I climbed in with her and told her she had been very brave at the hospital.

"I didn't like it," she said. Grace was a tough kid, stoic, wry, strong-willed. She had defended herself against her big brother and schoolyard bullies. She stamped her feet when she got angry. She held her ground. But in that moment, her lip trembling, she looked vulnerable and small. "I've never been in a hospital," she said. "And I didn't like it."

Even as I assured her that she would probably never be in a hospital again and tried to get her excited about having a broken arm—all those signatures!—I couldn't shake the feeling that something was wrong. I stayed with Grace until she fell asleep, stroking her hair and kissing her head, the way a mother would. As it turned out, her sleep that night was fitful, the arm aching, the codeine they'd prescribed not helping very much.

In the morning, I declared a holiday for Sam, and set about getting our bed ready for Grace. She would be waited on all day, I decided. She could watch television and color and drink her milk, all from our bed. I fluffed pillows and I opened windows to let in the warm air of another beautiful spring day. Once she was settled, I thought, I would bake her some of the peanut butter cookies she liked so much. Maybe tomorrow she would even be ready to go to school.

That morning after Grace broke her arm, before I could do any of these special things, she spiked a fever of 104. My frantic calls to the doctor who had treated her in the ER, the pediatric orthopedist she was scheduled to see later that week, and the hospital all went unanswered. By noon, I was frightened enough to call our own doctor, who suggested we go straight to the ER. Except for whimpering, Grace was unresponsive as I carried her to the bathroom and then into the car. That feeling that something was very wrong had abated a bit the night before, but never left completely. Now it was growing.

Like all mothers, I had nursed my children through fevers and bruises and a variety of typical childhood ailments. Both of them had had pneumonia; both had a history of allergy-related asthma. I had doled out antibiotics and bandages, and taught them how to use an inhaler of Albuterol. I had cleaned up my share of vomit and blood. But all of it fell within the realm of normal kid stuff. Suddenly I was thrust into a new place where doctors murmured together and turned their frowns on me.

I abandoned the car in the drop-off in front of the hospital and raced into the emergency room, Grace in my arms. The looks on the faces of the triage team let me know I was already considered a hysterical mother. Bored by something as mundane as a high fever, they gave Grace Tylenol and an exhausted doctor took notes through yawns about her symptoms. Lorne had gone to the police station to file a report on his stolen car, so once the doctor and nurse shuffled away, I was alone in a treatment room with Grace.

I kept calling her name, and she would struggle to open her eyes and focus them on my face before drifting off again. Was it the codeine making her like this? Or something else? I had asked the doctor, but he had declared her simply "sleepy." In the hospital next door to this one, where Grace was born, the maternity nurse had dubbed her the same thing: a sleepy baby. Even as a newborn, she would nurse happily, snuggle close, and sleep for hours. The word had seemed soft and special then. Now it terrified me. She hadn't had a dose of codeine in more than six hours. Shouldn't it be wearing off? But the doctor had only grinned and shrugged. "She sure is sleepy," he'd reiterated.

Alone with my little girl in her flowered baby doll pajamas, I called her name over and over, until in a lull of quiet, she went into a full-blown seizure. I had never seen one before except on television, but I knew what was happening and ran out of the room screaming for help. My friend Amy, the mother of a chronically ill child, once told me that the halls of hospitals are filled with mothers' screams. Now I added mine to all of the others. For the first of what was to be many times over the next thirty-six hours, doctors and nurses pushed me out of the way and refused to let me near my daughter. And I fought my way back to her, asking them what was going on, what was happening.

After the seizure stopped and Grace slept, the doctor asked me questions, his voice slightly befuddled. Did she always have febrile seizures? How much Tylenol had she had? How much codeine? At each response, he shook his head. Finally, he told me she would get a chest X-ray to check for pneumonia, a spinal tap to check for meningitis, and a CAT scan to check for brain injury. Ridiculously, I tried to decide which terrible scenario would be best.

"A little girl in her class has strep," I told him.

The doctor shook his head. Her throat, he said, didn't look at all like a strep throat.

When Sam was a year old, we'd had a scare with him while I was visiting friends in New York City. That morning, Sam—usually an early riser—was still asleep when I woke at nine. Found him in his portable crib, limp as cooked spaghetti. Without thinking, I ran across the street to Saint Vincent's Hospital, where they started IV antibiotics and then did tests. It turned out he was hypoglycemic. But standing in this hospital emergency room now, I remembered how they had done the same tests: chest X-ray, spinal tap. All he had needed was a big drink of orange juice, but they'd kept those antibiotics going.

"Maybe you could start her on antibiotics?" I suggested.

The doctor shook his head again. "We don't even know what she's got," he said, "so how would we know what to give her?"

I started to tell him about Sam all those years ago, but he was wandering out, puzzling over Grace's chart. My husband returned and I told him what had happened. We followed the gurney to X-ray, and to the CAT scan. We held Grace's hand while they performed an echocardiogram, and again while an intern fumbled through the spinal tap. By now Grace was awake, though far from alert. "Typical after a seizure," a nurse said, patting me on the back in a way that let me know I was officially considered a pain in the neck.

Test results began trickling in. Her heart was fine. Her brain was fine. Her lungs were fine. I glanced at Grace. She wasn't fine, that was clear to me.

"So what is it?" I kept asking, and the doctor and the trail of nurses and even new doctors all shrugged, unconcerned.

With each new face, I told the story again: the lethargy the day before, the fever, the seizure, the way she still wasn't acting like Grace. Everyone nodded and offered an explanation. Now she was acting this way because of the seizure. Or because of the fever which, a nurse proudly pointed out, was almost normal.

But every time I said "Grace" and watched her struggle as if from a long distance to answer me, my worry grew.

The doctor came in, yawned, and declared her fine. "We've got a room waiting for her upstairs," he said. "She'll go home in the morning and you'll set up a follow-up with a neurosurgeon."

"A neurosurgeon?" I said.

"Just protocol," he said, waving his hand. "She's fine. Just sleepy."

What mother doesn't want to hear that her child is fine? I imagined sleeping on the hard vinyl hospital chair in her room and waking up with her fever gone, her blue eyes sparkling again. Tomorrow we would go home, and I would feed her chicken with stars soup, and we would talk with great relief about our scary hours in the hospital.

Once Grace was settled into a bed, a chipper nurse came in and told us where to find videos and snacks.

"Do you want a Popsicle?" she asked Grace.

Again, Grace seemed to work very hard to focus on the question.

"You love Popsicles," I said, my voice still sounding desperate. "Grape?"

While the nurse left to get one, I watched Grace's temperature start to go up.

"Her fever's high again," I told the nurse when she returned.

"I'll get her some Tylenol," she said cheerfully.

In the moment before she came back, I climbed onto the bed with Grace. The Popsicle was melting down her small hand, and she had too big a chunk in her mouth.

"Be careful," I told her. "You have to chew that, sweetie."

She looked at me, and her baby blue eyes looked dark. Strange.

"Grace?" I said.

She managed to say "Mama."

"Honey?"

Again, that rising panic. Again, my shouting for help.

"Mommy's right here," I said, worried that another seizure was coming. Or some unnamable thing that was even worse. "I love you, Gracie. I'm right here."

From that distant place, she traveled again. "I love you, Mama," she said.

My husband appeared with our friend, a doctor at the hospital next door.

"Grace," I said, "it's Andy Green. Say 'hi.'"

Andy looked at Grace, and I saw his face change. He turned abruptly and walked out to the nurses' station. I saw him on the phone there, and then I saw him talk to Lorne and the two of them started to cry.

"Something is very wrong with Grace," Andy said. He had known her since she was born, had known us even longer.

"What do you mean?" I said. I think I was screaming again.

A medical team from the ICU burst into the room then, pushing me away from Grace. A doctor was screaming orders. Nurses were keeping me away. And I was yelling to Grace, "I'm here! I'm here! I'm here!"

Grace was dying. That's what they told us. No one knew why. They only knew that they had to fight to keep her alive. Part of a mother's job is to take care of her child, to keep her safe, to protect her. But here I had to *fight* to do any of those things. I fought to stay in the room with her. I pushed away the nurses who tried to keep me away from my little girl, who lay naked and vulnerable on a gurney under bright lights, her blood pressure rising and falling erratically, her heartbeat irregular. What did I know of the things she needed to live? Nothing. I only knew this: I had to be with her every minute. I had to let her know that I had not abandoned her.

At one point a surgeon came to tell us that they needed to operate on Grace's arm, but she was too fragile to move to an operating room. Instead, they were going to do it right there in the ICU. I left the room then, and lay on the floor at its doorway, as if Grace could smell me out there. Periodically, the door would open and a nurse would report to me that Grace was hanging in there. I don't know how long this went on, but eventually it was over and I was allowed back in. But all I could do was press my lips to Grace's ear and tell her I was there and that I loved her. Then I would beg her to live.

No one told me anything unless I asked questions. So I asked and asked and asked. What was that machine? That new IV? That lab test? Was she better yet? Once, after the doctor shook her head no, Grace was not any better, I moaned, "What is going on?"

The doctor said, "She has strep. But not in her throat. In her bloodstream."

"Strep?" I repeated. "When did you find that out?" I could hear my own voice telling each new doctor and nurse that a kid in her school had strep throat. I could still picture that doctor telling me she didn't have strep. But then something settled in me.

"Strep?" I said again. "So you can treat it." I thought of all the times I had administered amoxicillin to both of my children and how quickly they recovered.

"The antibiotics are treating that, but it's ravaged her organs now." She went on to explain how no one understood why the same bacteria that caused strep throat sometimes mutated into this virulent, usually deadly form.

"The broken arm," I managed, remembering how I had almost kept her home that day.

But the doctor was already dismissing me. That lethargy in the morning was the beginning of her getting sick. The incubation was two to five days. She probably got it some time over the weekend. Our weekend had been a flurry of birthday parties for her friends and even one for a family friend. I thought of all the people she had hugged and touched, the mats at the gymnastics party and the farm animals at the other one. Somehow I had let this horrible thing come to her. I had not done my job. I had not protected her.

Now her life was in the balance, and all I could do was whisper to her and smooth her hair. All I could do was watch her, watch the people caring for her, stay alert for any changes at all. In my vigilance, I saw the blood pooling around her, soaking the sheets and turning her hair pink.

"Is this okay?" I asked. "All this blood?"

I tried to remember how much blood we had in our bodies. But the sight of so much coming from Grace made me not want to remember.

Activity increased again. A doctor explained that her stitches from the operation hadn't held. Nurses cleaned up what they could, but the room kept the smell of rust in the air.

Then, like a gift, like magic, everything began to change. Her skin turned pink. Her liver function improved. Her kidneys were strong. The lights were finally dimmed and the sense of desperation that had hung over Grace, over all of us, lifted. Nurses started to smile at us and tell us what to expect over the next few days and weeks. The surgeon returned to tell us he was going to move her to an operating room and try to save her arm. This was the first I had heard that she might lose it. But my surprise quickly faded into resoluteness. Grace was getting better. Some day in the near future she would be back home with us.

Lorne brought in her favorite Beatles tape, *One,* and played it for her. The anesthesia was reduced so that we could talk to her.

"Do you feel sick?" Grace nodded.

"Do you know that I am here?" She nodded again.

"Do you know that I love you?" A smile and another nod.

She needs rest, we were told, and so the anesthesia was increased again. They talked about weaning her from the ventilator, how that would work, what to expect. They told us that with all the fluids that would get pumped into her, she would look like the Michelin Man. We laughed, giddy with hope.

The second surgery went well. The doctor looked at us and said, "Your daughter is going to make it."

I had not slept in almost forty-eight hours. Relief and exhaustion took over. A nurse brought in a reclining chair, a blanket. Everyone was so goddamned happy. I kissed Grace and told her I was right here, that I was just going to sleep for a little while. I told Grace that I loved her.

My daughter's blond hair has turned pink from blood.

"You can wash it tomorrow," a nurse tells me.

I can't seem to stop playing with Grace's hair, smoothing it, rubbing the fine pink strands between my fingers.

The nurse has me by the elbow now, urging me firmly away. "Tomorrow," she says again. "You'll see. That comes right out."

I let her bring me to my bed for the night. I let her pull a blanket over me. I close my eyes.

Two hours later, I wake up to noise and lights and a return of that frantic desperation. Jumping to my feet, I knock over the recliner, screaming.

A nurse looks at me and says, "We're losing Grace."

A doctor shouts for someone to get the mother out of here.

They do get me out, but I can't stop screaming. Not while they run in and out of the room. Not while they pound on my little girl's chest with such force that I almost have to look away. Not while the intercom calls for cardiology, telling the entire hospital that Grace Adrain is in cardiac arrest. I scream and I scream, as if my little girl can hear me: "Gracie!" I scream. "I'm here! Gracie! Mama's here!"

Once they tell me she is dead, and I run screaming down the hall and relatives race from the waiting room to my side, I want nothing more than to go home. But the nurses want me to do things. They want me to give her a bath. They want me to paint the bottoms of her feet pink and press them onto paper to preserve her footprints. They want me to decide whether or not to consent to an autopsy. I look at my daughter and she is dead, and it is freaking me out. I feel like I should be doing something brave and maternal, like cradling her in my arms. But I just want to go home. I want to get Sam at his friend Isabella's and take him in my arms and carry him home with me.

"Her hair," a nurse is saying. "You never got to wash it."

I look down again and there it is, the pink, bloodstained hair.

"Do you want to wash it now?" the nurse says.

I shake my head. My legs are shaking up and down, trying to take me away. An incredible thirst overtakes me and I start to drink the bottles of Poland Spring water that a friend delivered a million years ago when Grace was getting better. I drink one after the other, but somehow they just make me thirstier. I am on a desert. I am not in my own country anymore, where little girls don't have blood in there hair, where they don't die. I keep drinking water and trying to escape this new place where I have inexplicably landed. But I just keep getting thirstier.

"Do you want more time with her?" a nurse is asking.

I know that the answer is supposed to be yes. I look at my daughter and realize that I have failed her. Despite all of the things I have done since the New Year's Eve when she was conceived, right through these terrible few days when I screamed myself hoarse trying to help her and stay with her and take care of her, despite all of these things, she is five years old and she has died. I have somehow let her down.

"Your shirt," the nurse says to me.

I put it on so long ago that I have to remind myself what shirt I am wearing. It is a pale blue cotton shirt, baggy fitting with short sleeves and pale blue buttons.

"There's blood all over it," the nurse says, pointing.

I look down and see that Grace's blood is splattered all over the front of my shirt. I wonder at which point in this horrible nightmare did this happen?

The nurse grabs my arm. She holds on tight. "Don't wash it," she tells me. "Don't ever wash it. Take it off and put it away just like that."

"Okay," I tell her.

Eventually I leave that room, that ICU, that hospital. Eventually I get my son and we all go back home, all of us exhausted and heartbroken and stunned. I undress to climb into bed with what is left of our family. I unbutton the shirt. I fold it carefully and place it on the high shelf in my closet. Time passes. Months, then years. Still, I cannot help feeling that I let Grace down somehow. Concerned friends and family members and even therapists remind me of my vigilance. They shake their heads and tell me that they would not have even taken her to the hospital for that fever. They remember how I wouldn't leave her side to take their worried calls, how I slept on the hospital floor just to be close to her.

I have come to ease up on myself a little. I *was* vigilant; I *was* demanding; I *was* a good mother. But isn't a mother's job to protect her child? Perhaps if everything hadn't happened so fast, if I'd had time to understand all we were about to lose, I would not feel such regret, such a maternal lacking. There are days when I am almost there, but never all the way.

Even now when I open that closet I see the pale blue shirt high on its shelf. I touch it lightly with my fingertips. Beside it is Grace's brush, her fine blond hair still tangled in it. They remind me of the lands where I have traveled: That happy long ago one where my daughter held my hand tight and we walked through it together; that bloodstained place where I could only scream for help and smooth my daughter's hair and whisper to her to live; and this new land, foreign and empty. This land is post-apocalyptic. I wander it uncertain of what to do here, who to tend. My hand is empty, unsure where to rest. Someday I will unfold that pale blue shirt and I will follow the map of my daughter's blood. But not yet. Not yet.

the vital role

AMANDA FORTINI

In my early twenties, I returned from a writers' conference in Belize not with the improved compositional skills and new professional contacts I had hoped for, but with a debilitating tropical illness. The bug announced itself with an alarming ferocity, an intruder kicking down the door of my body's defenses. Thirty-six hours after my return, I fell into bed with muscle aches, joint pains, fever, bloating, gastrointestinal upset, and a rogue nausea that refused to reside in my gut, as queasiness usually does, and instead seemed to range about my entire body. For days I alternated between delirious, febrile sleep and frantic dashes to the bathroom. Finally, after an agonizing week, the siege appeared to be over; the mysterious sickness receded. Ten days later, it returned with even greater violence before once again departing. During the next few months the illness would follow this pattern, attack and retreat, attack and retreat, leaving me increasingly unwell with each incursion. Its martial tactics struck me as a fitting metaphor for the war evidently taking place between my immune system and whatever was roiling inside me.

At some point during those first fitful months, the acute flare-ups settled into the long, slow smolder of chronic illness. The "spells," as I had taken to calling them, still arrived with bimonthly regularity, but they had become much less distinct, muffled by the white noise of incessantly clamoring symptoms. At work, my boss began to question my frequent forays to the bathroom, as though I might be indulging a cocaine habit or an eating disorder instead of answering his phone. The tissues around my elbows, knees, wrists, ankles, and hips ached almost constantly. It hurt to cook, to type, to carry groceries. The nausea was relentless, so overwhelming that I often found myself locked in bathroom stalls around Manhattan, dry-heaving. (I became an expert on the whereabouts and cleanliness of the city's limited public restrooms.) Eventually, the illness bludgeoned me into heavy-limbed exhaustion. I managed to drag myself to my magazine job each day and then stumbled home to collapse into bed. If this was a war, it was a war of attrition, and my resources were dwindling.

I saw doctors, and, as the illness progressed and these initial doctors failed to diagnose it, more doctors. Most of the doctors shrugged and threw up their hands. Some of them dismissed me as neurasthenic, neurotic, and, given my dramatic weight loss, possibly anorexic. A few arrived at untreatable syndromes and talked of managing symptoms. Several months after my return from Belize, I learned that others who had attended the conference had also fallen ill, likely from a banquet served to us the final night, and a few had remained so. Given the relative impotence of Western medicine when faced with tropical disease, it would be nearly a year before I was diagnosed, another year before I was properly treated.

But this is not the story of that illness, its bizarre origins, its impossible diagnosis and obscure treatment. The illness is just the background to the story I want to tell, a story about the emotions that illness, particularly chronic illness, provokes in its sufferers and those who care for them—the anger, the anxiety, the jealousy, the fear, the generalized dysfunction. Perhaps I have told you all this by way of defending myself: *How can you blame me for my stupidity, my dependency, my bad behavior? I was so sick, so sick.* Because, difficult as it is for me to relate, this is the story of one peculiar relationship that sprung from the diseased soil of one peculiar illness. It is a story that arose from a perfect confluence of needs: one person's desperate need to be cared for and another's equally urgent need to care. It is the story of J.

The second time J. appeared in my life I had been sick for nearly two months. I felt exhausted and encumbered, as though I were trying to keep pace with the crowd while dragging an enormous suitcase full of rocks behind me. At this point, I was still attempting to live according to the city's hectic rhythms: long days at work, late nights out, weekend days spent rushing through errands. It was during one of these weekend after-noons that I spotted J. ferrying a boxed cake through the produce section at Dean & DeLuca.

She was impossible to miss. Her dyed platinum blond hair had black, peekaboo roots left naked for people to see. She wore dark prescription sunglasses always, day and night, rain and shine. She favored the shortest of short skirts—minis that rode high on her thighs and showed her panties when she bent over—paired with black opaque tights and towering plat-form boots, no matter the occasion or weather, and during a season when neither of these items were considered chic. She was in her midforties, but her face, pale and free of lines, had that tight, pulled, frozen quality of women for whom staying young is a priority. The overall effect was that of an aging, unemployed starlet, still beautiful but down on her luck. It was an image I am now sure she cultivated.

I didn't know her well, but I was glad to see her. She had been among the group of students with me at the conference in Belize. We hadn't actu-ally conversed much during the trip, though I had been fascinated by her eccentric appearance and the clipped, affected way she spoke, without tonal modulation or contractions, and with a fondness for self-consciously formal phrases like "the thing of it is" or "in point of fact." I had also been shocked by the Dorian Gray–ness of her looks when I heard her mention, one night at dinner, that she had seen *A Clockwork Orange* in the theater as a teenager. That she was so much older than she appeared only added to her mystique.

In the months since I had returned from Belize, I had kept my illness a secret, mostly because I was afraid to admit, especially to myself, just how sick I was. When I felt too nauseated to go out with friends, I pleaded too much work. At work, when people asked about my weight loss, I lied that I had taken up jogging. Now, when J. asked me how I had been, there was somehow no question of lying: "I haven't been well." I told her about my aching joints, the dizziness, the pain gnawing its way through my in-testines, the nausea that no amount of Compazine could touch. Since I was convinced that whatever was wrong with me had its source in Belize, some part of me was hoping for a shred of information—something—that would allow me to unravel this mystery and get well. Perhaps, too, I felt I could be open with her because she had been in Belize with me; she was present when the sickness, invisible and insidious, had begun.

To my amazement, J. told me she had also been unwell, that she had the same biting pains I had (she pointed to either side of her lower abdomen), that her digestion was disturbed, that she was abnormally tired, that she had lost weight. I stepped back to look at her; she did look thin. She had thought it was stress, or possibly her ovaries. She had been to the doctor, had not gotten answers. And she *did* want to talk about it. But. She raised the small white box she held in her hand. Tonight she was having a party. It would be great fun! Did I want to come?

I am easily seduced by glamour. Like some tragic character from a Fitzgerald novel, I will overlook flaws of personality or lapses in judgment and morality if they are hidden beneath a comely, appealing surface. And so, that evening, nausea and intestinal pain be damned, I went to the party.

J. was living on Greene Street, in the smallish, secondary loft of a rich philanthropist who was also a well-known collector of photography. I didn't and still don't know the precise terms of their arrangement, but I know she was living there indefinitely, and for free. (In the dreamscape of one's early twenties, incongruous events or circumstances present themselves and it never occurs to one to ask the important questions, like why or how.) In the many days I later spent at that apartment, I never saw the philanthropist, who apparently lived in another downtown loft with his much younger fiancée. J. spoke of him as a patron. She said he wanted to support her art. At the time, all of it made perfect sense. Why not?

How to describe her art? She had self-published two novels, and this is how she came to attend the writers' conference in Belize, but these quirky little *romans à clef*—they were fictionalized diaries, really—were neither her primary mode of self-expression nor her most interesting creations. Her real artistic endeavors were the numerous parties she threw, the crazy ensembles she wore, the quasi-Warholian home movies she made with friends. She was especially fond of movies, making them, seeing them, talking about them, and she often said that a person should live as though

starring in the movie version of his or her life. In this, she was something
of a performance artist. Her existence was her art, her art her existence.
I think of her as a contemporary Clarissa Dalloway, whose creative impulses
saw their greatest expression in her grand soiree—the superlative mix of
summoned guests and the right choice of flowers. Or, perhaps less gen-
erously, as Edie Sedgwick, her life lived for the entertainment of others.
But I don't mean to trivialize J. Such people possess a tremendous sense of
vitality, an infectious sense of fun, and an unyielding sense of wonder even
in the face of the unpleasant or banal. They enchant the people around
them, and most of us, at least for a time, are more than willing to enter
into the alluring fantasy they create. Yet there is also a dark side to this
quest for the art in the everyday. If life is a work of art, one must always
be in search of (or in the process of creating) the moment of dramatic
flair. These, of course, tend to arise from the most extreme circumstances:
the situation poised on the edge of hysteria; the fragile, deteriorating
person.

   This is where I came in.

Our friendship happened, as some friendships do, first slowly and then
all at once. We talked on the phone a few times; she sent me her books;
we had dinner. And then I could not remember a time when she had not
been in my life. She made me feel like my formerly well self: smart, stylish,
full of fun. "That's genius," or "You're brilliant," she would say, and I admit
I tried to be my cleverest, wittiest self to provoke such praise from her.
About a month into our relationship, she began saying "I love you" when
we parted company or got off the phone. I thought it was odd the first
few times she said it, but still, I blurted out, "I love you, too." Later, I grew
to like it. In truth, I was happy to be drawn into her magical circle. There
was also something apt about the sentiment. The speed and intensity with
which our friendship took shape made it feel much like falling in love.

   She didn't have a job, which meant she was always, endlessly, available.
If I wanted to have dinner, she would meet me at a restaurant, usually
at an ultrahip place owned by the philanthropist, where we could get a
table and sometimes eat for free. If I needed to talk—about work, about

writing, about books, about men, but mostly, in those days, about feeling ill—she was there to listen and commiserate. I could call her at 4:00 A.M. if I wanted. And what excruciatingly self-conscious twenty-three-year-old doesn't want that?

She was full of idiosyncratic advice. Since she was more than twenty years older than I was, I credited her with a lifetime of experiential wisdom. She had one theory, a sort of watered-down Buddhism, that a universal energy thrums through all of us, and if we hurt any living thing, we hurt ourselves. The corollary to this, her version of karmic kickback, was that if one helped others this would redound to oneself. But many of her ideas had a dark, didactic edge. She frequently said that a bad job would cause disease, because a young woman she had known, someone who had worked for an irascible man at MTV, had died of stomach cancer. I should quit my job, she insisted, because it was stressful; never mind that it was prestigious. (It was stressful in the way that all jobs are, and I guess her failure to understand this explains why she didn't work.) Then there was the notion that got the most play, the one that filled me with a raw sense of panic: If you get sick and you live in Manhattan, you must leave, because it's impossible to get well in the city. It was for this reason, she pointed out, that she would be moving to Los Angeles.

Why did I take her word as gospel? I had no answers from the doctors, no diagnosis, and, without answers, no hope for improvement. I guess that her ideas, ridiculous and rigid and even superstitious as they seem now, gave me something to cling to.

Perhaps more than anything, our relationship was a welcome distraction from my increasing physical discomfort. If there was a party, never mind that I might have to lie down in the bathroom when I arrived, J. thought we should go. We could feel sick at home, or we could go out and try to forget about it. And since it was the fall of 1999, the last heady months before the new millennium, there were plenty of diversions to choose from. The mood of the city at that time was one of barely suppressed hysteria; everyone had Y2K predictions, and the impending end of the world seemed a good excuse for a party. This manic energy, this millenarianism, reflected our own sense of anxiety and possible doom. And yet according to J. there was no time to dwell: There was always an opening to attend, fresh conversations to be had, some sort of "art" to be made. By that time, I was leaving home only to work, but occasionally J. managed to convince me that I should pull my wan, emaciated self together and come along. "You look like a wraith," she would say, "but of course that's the style."

Then I grew sicker, and the party was over. For whatever obscure reason, likely owing to the inscrutable workings of our individual immune systems, J. bore up better under the illness. J. complained on occasion about her own disordered digestion and low energy. It upset her immensely; her health had always been solid, she often said, "like a rock." But she continued to fight it, even to improve, while I began to wither. I lost more weight. I ran fevers. I began to feel almost constantly lightheaded and dizzy. The nausea and dry heaves grew worse: more frequent, more intense. Many days, my brain felt blunted, my thinking fuzzy, as though someone had stuffed cotton in the crevices between its lobes. Other days, I was so tired I had to leave work early to lie down, even though I was an assistant at the magazine and I'd inevitably return to find my boss fumbling to retrieve voice mail and rummaging through the piles on my desk. Often, I fought through the fatigue and stayed at the office, sure that I was about to pass out. Eventually, I became so weak I had to take a leave of absence from my job.

Always, J. was there for me. She kept my apartment tidy. She entertained me with gossip and tales of her adventures in the world. I could no longer eat at restaurants because the rich food antagonized my nausea and caused my digestive symptoms to flare, but I was also too dizzy to stand to prepare a meal, so she shopped and cooked for me. Finally, she just moved into my tiny studio apartment.

We set up house. She brought a bag full of her nutty clothes and weird sunglasses and self-help books, and for several weeks, we spent every moment, waking and not, together. She ate at home with me instead of going out with her friends. She taught me yoga stretches and breathing exercises and made me perform them with her in the mornings, no matter how awful I felt. She taught me to cook vegetarian food—my apartment was so small you could see the stove from the bed—like brown rice, sautéed kale, meatless shepherd's pie, salubrious stuff that might help me get better. You could say she taught me to take care of myself.

Above all else, I was grateful for her presence. She kept pushing back her move to Los Angeles to stay with me—she invoked it constantly, as though to warn me, but I guess I thought it would never come to pass— and I could not fathom by what miraculous twist of fate this woman I had not known a mere six months earlier had decided to put her own life aside and care for me, but she had. We did not speak much about how un- tenable the situation was. I think we both knew that I would either have to get well enough to go back to work or else leave New York. In spite of this, I felt a sense of comfort, even something approximating security, during the days she was with me. I think I would have drowned in a black sea of fear and panic had I faced the experience alone. But J. let me feel that I was not and would never be alone. This is a patently false notion, but sometimes, especially during illness, empty hope is exactly the balm one needs.

With age comes an understanding, as Bob Dylan sings in "To Ra- mona," that "everything passes, everything changes," but at twenty-three, without the tempering influence of experience, I did not realize this. I was convinced that because I had been sick for months with no resolution in sight, I would always remain ill, and the thought made me despondent. Then, too, I had never experienced such extreme and prolonged bodily torment. The thought of what it might signify filled me with an almost suffocating dread. This, combined with the fear that the symptoms would never relent, proved a poisonous combination. I had once thought my- self a capable, if somewhat neurotic, young woman moving through the world, a woman in control, someone who would manage whatever life tossed at her. Yet here I was, a fearful, anxious, needy, querulous mess.

One night, the evening before I was to undergo a colonoscopy, I was in the process of the unpleasant, laxative-induced "clearing" that is required so the gastroenterologist has, as it were, a clean slate, when I be- gan to shiver uncontrollably. My mouth went dry. My pulse slowed to an abnormally low rate. I tried to stand up and the blood rushed to my feet. I saw blackness before my eyes. I wasn't cold, and I wasn't shaking out of any immediate fear—I had already had two colonoscopies, and knew they were nothing to be afraid of—but from something intensely physical, as though some deep, bedrock layer inside me had shifted and was beginning to crumble. I felt weaker than ever, and I knew my body was protesting all the procedures and trial courses of antibiotics ("maybe this will work"), all the stress, all the worry, all of it. J. sat on the edge of the bed and took my hand. She began to rub the soft, fleshy pad between my thumb and first finger. I didn't know it then, but this is an acupressure point, one that soothes pain, nausea, even migraines. It was the smallest of gestures. It was also just right.

Of course, it wasn't all smooth skating, and I could already sense the cracks in the ice. They were spreading; the pressure was taking its toll. We started to bicker. She pushed me to quit my job. She told me I should leave New York for Los Angeles. I resisted what I felt were her attempts at control. Minor irritations began to chafe until they created open sores. There was the afternoon that I fussed, for some reason I can't now fathom, about her wiping down my countertops with a paper towel. Later that day, I complained that she hadn't washed the kale well enough. She had only given it a hasty rinse; shouldn't she scrub it with a brush? Something in her broke. I saw her inhale, her chest expanding with anger. She lifted the heavy cast-iron pan in which she had placed the greens and smashed it against the stove. Then she grabbed the greens and, with a sharp jerk of her thin arm, tossed them on the floor of my tiny galley kitchen. As she walked past me, she yelled, "You might want to think about why you're still sick!" And she crashed her way out, slamming the door behind her.

One of the most trying aspects of being sick is being cared for, as counterintuitive and thankless as that may sound. Nothing makes a person feel out of control—and illness by definition is a loss of control—like having to cede it to another person. All the cooking and cleaning and being ministered to was, I felt, turning me into a whiny, overgrown baby. She might as well have been wiping my bottom, I felt that uncomfortable. And I'm certain, when I think about it today, that this is exactly what she felt like she was doing.

As it happened, I was the one who had to move, and this is what finally let the air into the claustrophobic habitat we had created. My lease
ended, and the landlord didn't want to renew, so I hastily found an apartment through a friend. This impending change created an atmospheric
shift, invisible yet palpable, and J. took it as her signal to move on as well.
She arranged for her ex-husband, an affable and apparently obliging guy,
to come help me pack. He arrived with a CD by some pianist whose
name I've now forgotten, a box of Centrum Echinacea, and a book of tai
chi exercises. He told me J. had trained him well.

J. also arranged to borrow a friend's apartment, where she could stay
until her flight left, and I until my studio became available. (How did she
manage it? I was convinced that if she wanted a castle in France she could
find someone willing to lend her one.) With my apartment packed and
the boxes in storage, we rode uptown in a taxi together. When we arrived,
J. put sheets on the foldout couch where we'd sleep, filled the cabinets
with health food (rice cakes, canned beans, and the like), rented some
movies. At this point, with neither one of us working, we were living on
credit, charging even our groceries.

What especially bound me to her in those days, what I feared I would
miss most when she left, was the confidence we shared. J. was the only
person I could really talk to about being sick. For my friends, my cowork-
ers, even for most of my family, I painted the problem with the broadest
of strokes. This was partly out of pride. I was ashamed of being so ill, and
worried that others might view me as somehow tainted. But it was also
impossible to articulate the tangle of fleshly symptoms and spiritual anguish I was experiencing. Language is hopelessly inadequate to describe
physical suffering. "English," Virginia Woolf writes in her essay "On Being Ill," "which can express the thoughts of Hamlet and the tragedy of
Lear, has no words for the shiver and the headache. It has all grown one
way. . . . [L]et a sufferer try to describe a pain in his head to a doctor
and language at once runs dry. There is nothing ready-made for him." A
headache is a headache is a headache. The word conveys little about the
quality of the pain, and nothing about the emotional distress pain nearly
always produces. Words like "searing" or "burning" or "gnawing" (the one
I frequently employed) leave vast prairies of feeling unaddressed. There is

only metaphor or analogy to fall back on, but without a familiar referent, these too lack meaning. The inability to express the experience of illness with any degree of precision creates an immense divide between the sick and the well.

It also means that illness is by and large a boring subject, and anyone who discusses it is considered a bore, too. Alphonse Daudet, a popular nineteenth-century French novelist who suffered and died from syphilis, writes about the tedium of illness in *In the Land of Pain,* a short, impressionistic chronicle (compiled from notes he made for a book he never wrote) of his increasing debilitation. "Pain is always new to the sufferer," he writes, "but loses its originality for those around him. Everyone will get used to it except me." For the sufferer, each new agony produces fireworks of a different color, but for the person who hears about it, it all sounds like the same noise. Even if your head or your joints ache more or less or differently, they still ache. Nothing, it seems, has changed. The young are particularly guilty of this sort of impatience— *"You're still sick?"*—and at the time, the majority of my friends were young.

This served to isolate me, and to draw me closer to J. With J., I could say I "felt nauseated" or was "having those pains again" and not only did she listen with interest, she essentially knew what I meant. In my mind, she was the only one who understood what I was going through; why should I bother to explain my problems to anyone else? The unusual circumstances of the situation—the fact that we both had the same illness— meant that this sentiment, which would normally have been juvenile in the extreme, a kind of adolescent soul-mate syndrome, was not so unreasonable. And yet in creating this isolation of perfect empathy, I also created a wind tunnel filled only with her air. Since there were no countervailing currents to offset her, J. came to hold far too much sway.

Late one afternoon, a few days before she was to depart, we sat on the couch in the borrowed apartment, eating some rice cakes and watching a snowstorm blanket the city with its white, unforgiving presence. J. turned to look at me.

"You have to leave New York."

"Huh?"

"You'll die if you stay here."

"I won't *die*."

"If you stay, you'll never get out."

By then, I had a sense that she ran toward the dramatic, but I also knew what she meant.

"Come to Los Angeles," she said for the umpteenth time. "It's sunny. You'll get better. And you can live with me."

And then, finally, it was time for her to go. My memory of her leaving is strange. It is dark. I am in the foldout bed and she is standing over me, like a mother tucking her child in for the night. Can this possibly be right? Did her flight depart early in the morning? Did I not bother to get up? Of course the image, whether real or imagined, is symbolic. "Do you think it's going to be all right?" I ask, looking up at her.

"It's going to be just fine," she answers. I do not believe her.

For a long time, I liked to think that my total physical collapse was unrelated to her departure. In fact, the breakdown did have a medical basis: I had acquired a super-bacteria, the drug-resistant sort you're supposed to watch out for in hospitals, from being treated too aggressively and frequently with antibiotics; the resulting infection had left me so feverish and fluish that I couldn't be out of bed for more than a few hours at a time. But it's also true that my immune system waved its white flag not two weeks after she had left. What can I say?

In the end, I went to Los Angeles. I didn't know what else to do. Los Angeles seemed to hold at least the possibility of a turnaround—the pale mirage of a sun-filled, healthy new life.

J. picked me up at the airport. The five-hour flight had drained me, and I was dying to get into a bed. She had a man with her, thirtyish and skinny. His name was Mattie, he told me, as he gave my hand a limp shake.

He said very little after that. J., meanwhile, never stopped talking. I'd be alone this time. She was staying with Mattie now. She didn't tell me on the phone because she wanted me to come. The thing of it was, they wouldn't be that far away, just a twenty-minute car ride. I could call them if something happened or I needed anything or I wanted to go somewhere. But they were sort of busy right now. They were making a movie together. And on and on. I didn't quite understand this sudden shift in allegiance; I listened and said nothing in response.

Her apartment was far into East Hollywood, in a neighborhood that has only recently begun to gentrify. We walked through the courtyard around which two levels of tiny apartments wrapped. There was a dirty-looking swimming pool with leaves and grass floating in it that reminded me of the depressing little pool in the opening scene of *The Karate Kid*. The apartment itself had a kind of Astroturf for carpeting, green and nubby and scratchy to the touch. In the main room, there was no furniture except for a folding chair and a table on which an old desktop computer sat. There wasn't any furniture in the bedroom, either. "Where do you sleep?" I asked her. She pointed to the yoga mat rolled up on the floor.

"Don't you use a pillow?" I looked around for one.

"I find I don't really need one."

I walked around the corner, back into the main room, to look at the corridor of a kitchen. There was no refrigerator.

"How do you eat? I mean, where do you keep your food?"

"I generally ride my bike to the market each morning and buy food." I didn't have a bike, and I certainly didn't have the wherewithal for daily rides to the market.

"We can just drive, can't we?"

"Well, right now I don't have a car." Her car had broken down the week before but she had forgotten to mention it. Mattie had been driving her around. She was trying to get her sister to lend me some jalopy she had sitting in her driveway, but no one was sure if it would start.

As I stood there surveying the all but empty apartment where I'd be staying, I had to make an effort not to gasp audibly in disbelief. *This* was not a place to get well. I'd had no idea she lived such a down-to-the-bone existence. Suddenly all the borrowed apartments, the shuttling between places, the willingness to stay with me, made a sort of sense. *What had I been thinking to come here? How had I been so naïve?*

"We'll see you tomorrow." They walked out.

The first night in her apartment, I felt trapped, a prisoner driven half-mad by her stark, narrow cell. The neighborhood wasn't safe after dark, so I couldn't leave. The apartment didn't have heat, and California in January is surprisingly chilly. There was no diversion: no television, no radio. And since there were neither pillows to lean on nor a couch nor a bed to sit on, it was nearly impossible to read. I sat on the Astroturf carpeting with my back against the cold wall and flipped through a book she had lying on the floor, something about vibrational medicine. In a kitchen cabinet I found a box of cereal and polished it off dry. I rolled the yoga mat out and tried to sleep.

J. came to pick me up for lunch the next day—after the cereal was gone, there was nothing left in the kitchen save a plastic bag containing a few stale clumps of granola—and as soon as we got into the car I began to lob my complaints. (I had, after all, just spent the night on a yoga mat.) I was tired. My neck hurt from sleeping without a pillow. My back ached from the yoga mat. I was starving. I had no car. The apartment was freezing.

J. slammed her foot on the brake. My body lurched forward. I wasn't wearing a seat belt. I threw my hands out in front of me to stop my head from smacking the dashboard.

"You know," she screamed, turning to face me as we sat there, the car idling, in the middle of the street. "The hole in you is so deep I could throw my entire body in and that wouldn't be enough!"

A feeling of tightness spread over my chest, and deeper, into my lungs. I couldn't talk, could barely breathe. Playing the part of the big baby she was telling me I was, I started to cry.

Was she right? Had I been that awful?

What had I expected from her? Any armchair psychologist would have gone your basic Freudian route and said that I was trying to make her a substitute for my absent mother, who lived in Chicago, who was distracted by her own life's drama, and, when it came to my illness, preferred a laissez-faire approach. (For the first time in the sixteen years since she and my father divorced, my mother was dating, and she was on the cusp of getting engaged.) Just as a child expects her mother to be responsible for her needs, the argument would go, I had expected J. to fulfill my own. This may have been partly true, but it was also true that I had not wanted from her anything she had not offered. And it wasn't, of course, the yoga-mat bed or bare apartment that had upset me. Those were just surrogates for the abandonment I felt. I had come to Los Angeles because she had promised me something—a safe, comfortable place to stay, not to mention her companionship—and she had, without warning, pulled that soft, plushy rug out from under me and replaced it with, well, Astroturf. In doing so she made it clear, intentionally or not, that not only did I have to take care of myself, but that we are all ultimately alone. It was a sobering realization, even more so for the unceremonious way it was delivered. Yet however dishonest and indelicate J. had been with me, I had been equally unfair to her. I had expected her simply to *be there,* to keep me company, to prop me up when I was feeling especially sick or down. I had expected her to make me forget about the enormous, intractable black hole of a problem at hand, if not actually to fix it. I guess I had expected her to distract me—like some court jester, some dancing monkey—from my symptoms.

But as much as I craved it, there was also something insufferable to me about her excessive caretaking, her constant *thereness,* for lack of a better word. I had begun to realize that I didn't know much at all about this woman who had bound up her life with my own. It seemed that her bottomless empathy and her empty apartment were not wholly unrelated. I think I had—we both had—reached nearly the point of suffocation. And perhaps my complaining was at its root a reaction to that. Put simply, I provoked the fight to push her away. "Here we go alone and better like it so," Virginia Woolf writes. "Always to have sympathy, always to be accompanied, always to be understood would be intolerable." This is the great paradox of being cared for; as much as you want someone there with you, you also, in the end, don't.

. . .

We didn't see much of each other after that. I dipped into my meager savings and rented a car, a boxy white Honda. I knew I couldn't yet hold down a demanding job, which meant I also couldn't afford to return to New York. I figured I had a free place to stay, austere as it was, and that I might as well make the most of it. I went to a discount mattress store and bought a mattress and box spring and bed frame for $300. I found an acupuncturist in the Valley who took my insurance, and began to see her several times a week. Nights I lay in the apartment in a state of half-sleep listening to the neighbors through the cardboard walls, playing video games and then, as though the games were foreplay, having sex. Days I aimlessly drove the freeways, like Maria from *Play It As It Lays*. (Somehow, feeling the wheel beneath my hands, knowing my life depended on its steadiness, began to restore my sense of control.) Often, as I drove, I grew so tired I had to return home to lie down. I cried a lot. Many days I did not get out of bed. I was miserable, but I was also learning that most crucial adult lesson, obvious and yet so difficult to internalize—that life is full of discomfort, that it requires the endless doing of things you don't quite feel well enough to do. And at length, through some combination of time and rest and self-reliance and Chinese herbs, I started to regain my strength.

The end, when it came, played out as swiftly as the beginning. Late one afternoon I drove, for the first time, to visit J. at Mattie's house. He lived in a single-room apartment on the edge of Silver Lake, an arty neighborhood with an industrial feel. J. was hovering over the ancient stove, making vegetarian burritos. Mattie asked her for a cup of tea, and she filled the kettle and turned on the burner. He sat on the bed while she bustled about. The floor was the only other place to sit, so I stood to talk to them. Mattie wasn't working, but he was looking for a job, maybe as a writer's assistant. J. was helping him get things together. I asked Mattie about the sling he was wearing on his arm. He told me he had carpal tunnel syndrome. I asked him if it was from typing too much—at last, here was a topic over which we could connect—but he said no, it was from playing too much foosball at the local bar.

I arrived back at J.'s apartment to find a woman in her midtwenties sitting at the desk using the computer. Her inky black hair hung down her back in a tangled mass, and she wore scarlet lipstick that stood out brightly against her pale, freckle-dusted skin. Despite the wide-set prettiness of her features, her face had a hard, constricted appearance, particularly around her jaw, almost as though she kept it permanently clenched. There was the tension of recent recovery about her, a hypervigilant alertness. I had a sense she kept the chaos at bay by holding herself like a tightly balled fist.

"Um, hi?"

"Hi." She did not turn to look at me.

"Who are you?" I asked her, stepping nearer to the desk, as close as I could get to her field of vision.

"I'm V." Typing.

"May I ask what you're doing here?"

"J. gave me a key." Still typing.

"Oh?"

"She lets me come here sometimes to take baths."

I didn't know what to say to *that*—no, you can't have your bath?—so I tried to make small talk while she continued to check her e-mail.

"What does V stand for?" I was thinking Violet, maybe Victoria.

"Violence." She paused. "It was a name I got when I was a junkie and a prostitute." She turned to look at me. "Isn't J. the greatest?"

I agreed that she was.

"She saved my life."

In that moment, the past year came into a kind of sharp focus. It was as though I had been looking through the wrong end of a pair of binoculars and I had suddenly turned them around. Any lingering illusions I'd held that I was an exceptional case were quickly dispelled. Maybe she hadn't cared for me because she'd recognized someone worth caring for; maybe it had nothing to do with me at all. It appeared that I was just one in a series of fixer-upper projects. The idea was upsetting, but it also freed me of some of the embarrassment and guilt I felt about my wretched, undignified behavior. I realized, all at once, that as much as I had needed J., she had needed me, too.

I was reminded of the Ted Hughes poem "Fever," in which he writes about caring for an ill Sylvia Plath:

> *I bustled about.*
> *I was nursemaid. I fancied myself at that.*
> *I liked the crisis of the vital role.*
> *I felt things had become real.*

Was that it? The role made her feel necessary? Surely that was part of it. Still, it didn't seem that simple to me. Did tending to others anchor her life of perpetual drift? I thought of the loft on Greene Street, the borrowed apartment on the Upper East Side. It was almost as though she was in the business of caregiving—part of a large network of caring and being cared for in return. In a sense, there was something noble about it all. But it wasn't a way I could live.

I left her apartment the next day. I drained the last of my savings and rented an apartment in a temporary housing complex in Toluca Lake, just north of the 101 freeway. It was spring, pilot season in Los Angeles, and the building was full of child actors and actresses: kids screaming at stage mothers, stage mothers screaming at kids. It felt so appropriate.

Hardly two weeks had passed when, one afternoon, I stood up from the couch and turned my ankle over on itself. I heard a loud snap before I felt the excruciating shock of white-hot electricity shoot through my foot and up my leg. I knew immediately it was broken. On the verge of vomiting from the pain, I hoisted myself up onto the couch and called J. "I need to go to the emergency room. Can you take me?" I lay there, writhing inside, defeated. It was my right ankle. I would be unable to drive. Once again, I would be dependent on her.

That night, as I lay in bed with my ankle wrapped and my head swimming with Vicodin, J. arrived with groceries. This woman who ate only health food, who had taught me to eat it as well, had bought for me Häagen-Dazs ice cream, full-fat yogurt with the cream on top, potato chips, and several loaves of white bread. It was a transparently passive-aggressive act—it makes me laugh now, to think about it—but I couldn't blame her. Perhaps I had tested even her limits. Perhaps she thought I was ungrateful. Likely she knew I was leaving her; it was only a matter of time. I'm sure she also sensed that I had begun to judge her as critically as she had judged me. Whatever the reason, it was over. After she had gone, I called American Airlines and booked a ticket back to New York. "Is this a round-trip fare?" the operator asked.

"No," I said, some faint note of triumph in my voice, "it's one-way."

I limped around Manhattan, literally and figuratively, for a number of months. I went back to my job at the magazine. No one asked much about my time away, for which I was grateful, since I didn't want to talk about my strange cross-country interlude anyway. When I felt especially woozy, I closed myself in the conference room and put my head down to rest. Eventually, I found a diagnosis and treatment. I had a tenacious amoeba that had caused dysentery, and it required several rounds of noxious antiparasitic drugs to treat. In spite of the medicine, some of the symptoms never completely abated. The doctors say my intestines were damaged, likely permanently. I have to watch my health now like a protective parent hovering over a child. I tire more easily than I used to. I get sick more often than other people.

Two and a half years after I had left Los Angeles, I ran into J. I was eating alone at a table near the front window in an East Village vegetarian restaurant. She tapped on the glass; I waved her in. She ordered a salad and we chatted while we ate. She had moved back to New York. She was working part-time for a lawyer, living at a friend's place on the Lower East Side. We exchanged e-mail addresses and hugs.

Later that night I received an e-mail from her. "You looked beautiful as always today, but I am concerned about the color of your skin. Are you sick again?" I deleted the e-mail without responding. I would always be grateful to her, but I was no longer that girl.

. . .

I now live in Los Angeles, though I swore I'd never return. My life here is nothing like my initial sad sojourn. It is calm, stable. My apartment is furnished. I return to New York often for work, and, in a city full of people I'd love to see but never do—former classmates, old boyfriends—I run into J. with a frequency that would make me suspicious if I had a mind so inclined. We hug, exchange pleasantries. She is in nursing school, which seems to me right. She asks me how I am doing. I tell her I am well, even when I am not. We promise to get in touch, have dinner. We leave each other knowing we won't.

planet autism

SCOT SEA

L ose track of time on the phone, get distracted with the mail, day-dream over a cup of coffee—that's all it takes. The odor has finally made its way down the hall. When you see the balled-up pants and diaper on the floor you know you are too late. A bright red smear across the door, the molding, the wall. Turn the corner and the bedroom is a crime scene. An ax murder? In fact, it is only your daughter at her worst. (Worse than three days without sleep? Worse than ear-splitting screams that physically hurt, actually cause you to drop what you hold in alarm, compel you to shriek back at your delighted child who smiles at you sincere as a spring day?) Shit everywhere. Splashes of blood glistening like paint, black clots, yellow-brown feces, and a three-foot-diameter pond of vomit that your daughter stands in the middle of, a dog-eared copy of *Family Circle* in one hand, reaching for the TV with the other. She is naked except for stockinged feet, blood soaked up to her ankles. Hands dripping, face marked like a cannibal, she wears an expression of utter bewilder-ment: What's happened to me? Where am I? Is this good? Am I okay? There being nowhere to walk without stepping in some bodily emission, you throw bath towels down like a bridge to get to her.

Stripping her unavoidably stains you. A bloody handprint on the square of your back as she balances herself when you roll down her sop-ping stockings. You hope she touches nothing else but what does it matter as the bathroom remains appalling in spite of the previous cleanups: cabi-net handles encrusted with dried excrement, brown swipes on the light switch, corner of the mirror, shampoo bottle, Q-tips, ceramic figurines, curtain louvers. (Holiday guests take you aside to warn you of rodents in

unusual locations. Ancient turds in drawers, inside books. You thank them.
Apologize. Yeah, it's an ongoing problem.)

In the warm rain of the shower she proceeds to dig. She is excavating
for what remains of the impacted stool, hard as a French roll. This entire
episode, this habit, the result of some maddening control issue. The be-
haviorists, the gastroenterologists, the living-skills experts all suggest their
strategies and therapies and videos and diets and oils and schedules. Certainly she knows what you want—appropriate toileting. And there are
occasions when she does just that. Goes in, sits, finishes. This, maybe 5
percent of the time. Some huge, softball-size stool discovered in the toilet
bowl. You shout for each other and gaze in wonder as at a rainbow or falling star. That's how excited you are.

Get in the shower with your daughter. Wash her hair three times,
scrub her down, between the toes, everywhere. Take an old toothbrush to
her nails. Towel her down. Her hair, lightly—enough. Better stop. Know
how she hates that. Let the rest air-dry. Get her dressed. Diaper. Thank
God for extra large GoodNites. (Remember the college gal at Safeway
in her Birkenstocks and hemp sun hat: "Didja know," she must inform
you, "it's disposable diapers that are filling up America's landfills?") Next,
deodorant, sweat pants, the rest. Rewind the movies. Pop in her favorite
CD soundtrack (*Annie*) and program it for loop. Pull out a couple of old
Redbook magazines. Make sure all the doors are locked. Remember when
she wandered away, found in the middle of the street, a garbage truck
honking at her like she's some stray mutt.

Sooner or later, parents raising children with severe learning disabilities
receive the "Welcome to Holland" essay by Emily Perl Kingsley. It describes a couple planning the trip of a lifetime to Italy. They prepare and
study and learn everything they can about their cherished destination.
When their plane lands, though, an announcement: They have arrived in
Holland. Holland? They wail. We've dreamed all our lives of Italy. Italy is
where they want to be. Not here!

"But there's been a change in the flight plan," Kingsley writes.
"They've landed in Holland and there you must stay." New guidebooks,

a new language, a completely different group of people than those you hoped to meet. Worse still, "everyone you know is busy coming and going from Italy and they're all bragging about what a wonderful time they had there. And for the rest of your life you will say, 'Yes, that's where I was supposed to go. That's what I had planned.'"

Two hundred years ago most of these kids were tossed down the well or thumped against the fence post. It was either that or watch your own be torn to pieces by a coyote, or trampled to death in the corral, or find they had drowned in the duck pond or tumbled off a ledge or wandered off in a blizzard. If you were of an educated class, institutionalization became an option. A way out. There were always the few, though, whose pride or familial loyalty or stubbornness would not allow them to abandon such a child. Upright, determined mothers—mostly—who would rescue the idiot from the snow bank, from their husband's impassive grip, and nurse it and attend and teach the strange thing until the child might even say "hello" when ordered and carry a basket of eggs without stumbling.

"There's just something missing in his head is all. He be slow, like your Uncle Bert." The husband had grown up seeing three-headed lambs and bizarre carrots looking more like udders. He was aware of nature's imperfections. Sometimes it snowed in August. Sometimes the bread didn't rise. Best to throw out that mix. Best to keep the lines clean, the herds strong, purebred. But his wife refuses to push the runt away. Her husband, a man who shoots old mules and pulls out the dead weed and makes a Saturday night vest from the skin of a stillborn calf, has neither pity nor patience with the wife's indulgent efforts in the matter of the idiot. He will ignore the child. Like the lame piglet and the other orphaned stock following the wife around for a bottle, if she wants to put up with that, well, just keep 'em out of my way.

Autism. Auto, for "self," or "same." The tendency to view life in terms of one's own needs and desires . . . unmindful of objective reality (*Webster's*).

At one time a generic term applied to children navigating presocial orientation. Developmental psychologist Jean Piaget noted six-year-olds playing marbles as completely indifferent to rules, fairness, winners, losers. Two or more side by side yet no group norms emerged. Possibly each child played an entirely separate game. "[Their] relations to the world are autistic—determined largely by the wishes and preferences of the individual."

A tiny but multiplying percentage of seemingly healthy children persist in spurning socialization, cocooning themselves from human contact. Pediatric shrinks, at a loss, anoint the manifestation Serious Emotional Disturbance, later sanded down to "disorder." Enter Bruno Bettelheim, who postulates his infamous "refrigerator mom" theory. Everybody remembers this from Psych 101. How to explain these peculiar, silent, radically remote children? Normal and handsome in every other respect? Freudian, clearly. Cold, aloof mothers disdaining the maternal bond. Curiously, other siblings either below or ahead of the odd child have no complaints. Her ex-husband, his pride squashed, confused, castrated, weighs in for the prosecution: "That bitch was an iceberg! Kid wouldn't go near her." Of course, the kid wouldn't go near anyone. Anyone at all. (Autistic infants, it is believed, produce abnormally high levels of endorphins at birth; they receive no pleasure from bonding with their mothers and, by extension, ignore incentives for social interaction.)

Today, autism is recognized as a profound and mysterious neurological disorder characterized by certain behavior types and patterns of interaction and modes of communication. A spectrum disorder, in fact, encompassing so many symptoms that intake counselors, after exhausting considerations of Tay-Sachs, Fragile X, Klinefelter's and Turner syndromes, still categorize whole generations of two-year-olds as "other health impaired."

Media presentations emphasize the savants: the six-year-old Beethoven or the human calculator, or there, on Discovery Health, a teenage Rodin. The average autistic child, not excluding the savant, struggles with varying degrees of developmental retardation. They can operate the VCR but cannot button their coat. Have no interest in markers or crayons but will spend hours tearing paper, leaves, twigs into microparticles. Some are high-functioning—can read and speak, attend college, develop careers. Temple Grandin (autism's John Nash), a world-renowned authority on cattle psychology whose visionary stockyard designs have transformed one-third of the bovine and pork operations in this country alone, strolls through corrals of half-ton Herefords. They snort like grizzlies and paw the earth. She knows that one switch of their mighty heads would crush any man's clavicle, yet they allow her to walk among them, scratch their necks, communicate. The complexity of human interaction, however— reciprocity, *Romeo and Juliet*—remains as elusive to her as *colorless green ideas sleeping furiously.*

For better or worse, autism may be in the throes of its own fifteen minutes of fame. It's had recurrent cover stories in both *Newsweek* and *Time* and features on virtually all the TV magazine shows. Look, there's NFL star Doug Flutie frolicking with his autistic kid while shilling for a long-distance provider. Beck holds benefit concerts for autism research. A Nicholas Sparks potboiler concerned a missing child with autistic symptoms. A fictional senator on *The West Wing* filibusters Congress on behalf of his autistic grandchild. Our biggest stars share the screen with autistic protagonists: Richard Dreyfuss, Tommy Lee Jones, Bruce Willis, and Tom Cruise, most famously, supporting Dustin Hoffman's *Rainman,* a watershed entry in the MR Film Festival. Other screenings celebrate asylum romps—*King of Hearts; One Flew Over the Cuckoo's Nest; Awakenings; Quills; Girl, Interrupted*—films presenting madness as romantic, adorable or courageous—hence, *A Beautiful Mind.*

The movies prefer to apply the humanistic model to disability so that any attendant bleakness or the utter incomprehensibility of some conditions becomes only aberrant behavior immaterial to the subject's uniqueness as a human being. This same psychological model, however, views its members as basically rational, oriented toward a social world and motivated to getting along with others. But the autistic rarely makes adjustments to the world. Their own world remains self-generated and self-contained. Autism, as one text suggests, is "imagination self-determined." A world of, perhaps, pure imagination. Some autistic youngsters learn to sing before they ever speak. Others spin in place, their eyes closed, for hours, in their own encapsulated rave. Are they cursed, or are they angels among us? Poet Billy Collins asks,

> *Do they fly through God's body*
> *and come out singing?*
> *Do they swing like children from*
> *the hinges*
> *of the spirit world saying their*
> *names backwards and forwards?*
> *Do they sit alone in little gardens*
> *changing colors?*

Celestial metaphors do little to temper the exhaustion you struggle with as your daughter, still going strong at 3:30 A.M., cranks out her version of the diagnostic handbook for developmental disorders' greatest hits. This in spite of receiving her meds back, when? Seven that evening? Enough detox, compulsion blocker, and synapse stim to sober a junkie. But for some reason—full moon, diet, puberty?—her sleep patterns have been cross-circuited. The deeper into brutal night she marathons, the more wired, delirious, hypermanic she becomes. You have isolated yourself in her room. The same home-taped *Sesame Street* plays the same two and a half hours over and over. This, an integral part of the perseverative tic impelling her to clutch to her chest all manner of unrelated objects: a door stop, a bean bag, a ball of foil, a coaster, a hairbrush, a subscription card, a winter scarf. When she bends to pick up yet another item—a shoe—invariably the lot of it gets away from her, and you watch as the bundle spills to her feet. Dutifully, robotically, she gathers everything up again, dropping some, retrieving, dropping again like a bumbling vaudeville comic. You watch this fascinated, then impassioned, then with alarm *(what . . . the hell . . . is she doing?)*, then with dull acceptance. It is just the same scene from the same interminable clip on the late show from hell.

You doze. You wake, her hand on your face. Time to rewind the video. Surly with fatigue, you shove her aside as the school bully would some playground twerp. Clothes all over the floor. She's emptied her dresser, the closet. Inexplicable sculptures composed of sweaters pancaked with a book, then a stocking, a puzzle piece, an old moldy pretzel all constructed in mysterious, calculated intent. They dot the little room like totems, mushrooms, shrines amid a Japanese garden. You sit together as the VCR motor whines. Yoga on the TV—must be dawn. Beautiful bodies made of rubber on some tropical shore. Hey, they got nothing on your kid, whose quadruple-jointed limbs can do Cirque du Soleil moves. An hour later your wife wakes you. (What do you do without a partner? How is this possible alone? Sex . . . maybe a quick tumble whenever the kid sleeps. Jumping each other like scamps. Going at it. Then you notice your child standing in your bedroom, waiting. Standing there like Carrie, shiny red as a candied apple, wet footprints, dogs licking her legs. Coitus interruptus, anyone?) Sunlight streaming through the window. "Is she down?" you ask. "Is she asleep?"

"She's in the shower," your wife responds. "She got me up."

Daylight seems to click her down a few amps. She seems alert and ready for the day. A full circle has transpired and now, a familiar morning ritual. Calming, predictable. Breakfast. More pills. Hair. Teeth. Dressed. (Help your fifteen-year-old daughter on with her bra every morning and the female breast loses most of its mystery.) Get her on the special ed school bus. Now you must leave for work. Can't take any more sick days. So sleepwalk through the motions. Hope your reserves kick in. Take an early lunch. Doze in the car for an hour. Throw down three cups of mud stewing since morning. Limp till 5:30. Collapse at home. Sleep through midnight. Again, your wife wakes you. Yeah, she's still up, she informs you—napped two hours at school, cruising ever since. Your wife has clients tomorrow. She must crash. Time for your shift.

Men may be from Mars and women, indeed, Venus. But Planet Autism is where you reside now.

Doctors know everything. Doctors know squat. Hire an immunologist to pursue research your own internist finds superfluous. Ophthalmologists say don't bother with glasses—they'll never keep them on. Neurologists and psychiatrists prescribe truckloads of alchemy, names suggesting the moons orbiting this new world: Zyprexa, naltrexone, clonidine, ranitidine, trazodone. Some indeed become the magic pill. The miracle drug.

But getting there can resemble trial-and-error binges that would shrivel Hunter S. Thompson.

Ten years ago there were pediatricians who didn't know autism from the Ottoman Empire. Now it's the diagnosis du jour. An entire alternative health industry sprouts up around it. The usual suspects—some expert, or a blood chemist, or an Indonesian pharmacist—place an ad in *Prevention* magazine, publish a newsletter, hit the conferences, premiere a Web page, and before long a thousand parents are in line for facilitated communication, blue-green algae, auditory integration therapy, the secretin hormone, whatever. Maybe it will actually work? At least for a couple of weeks, maybe a month. If the guinea pig is your kid, she may demonstrate a promising response. Increased verbalization. Improved eye contact. Focused participation within some innocuous family activity. Then cruelly, predictably, her confused wiring, a permanent hard drive virus directs her biochemistry to countermand the positive results of the new substance, to develop, in effect, *immunity* to it. And so in time this latest exciting remedy becomes no more than an asterisk in the snake oil file.

Western medicine is on the defensive. The U.S. Department of Education reports a 900 percent increase in cases of autism since 1992. (Is anyone listening?) On C-SPAN, exhausted, terrified, furious parents vent their hopeless wrath during congressional hearings investigating claims that Big Pharma has ignored for years their belief that pediatric vaccinations precipitated their children's *acquisition* of autism. Was the mercury-based preservative contained in the vaccines—thimerosal—overwhelming the baby's premature immune system? A generation ago kids received these shots in measured intervals. Today, some infants get a concentrated cocktail so as to be done with it.

Bicker with, annoy, scream at, then finally threaten school administrators who want to dump your child in a room full of vegetables. Obtaining effective programs and services, you learn, is like squeezing water from wood. (What was the final straw that pushed Vermont Senator Jim Jeffords out of the GOP? Bush's refusal to increase federal funding for special education.) Fight like hell for the best curriculum, the best teachers.

Otherwise, you're just a rube swallowing input consisting of "sign here." Individualized Education Programs can be expensive. School districts will dig in their heels. Be reasonable, the administrators say. Fuck them. Demand everything. Let the band hold bake sales.

New Age pests, overdosed on media mythology, overhear you are the parent of an autistic child and, eyes aglow, pronounce, "Oh! And isn't that just a blessing?" In Wisconsin, storefront fundamentalists suffocate an eight-year-old autistic boy to death while attempting to "exorcise" his strange behaviors. Evangelicals offer how it is the world's collective sin that is to blame. Manifesting itself as suffering, wickedness, the mysterious afflictions that befall the innocent. Clueless neighbors, whose own children run wild, devoid of discipline, remark, "Yeah, our kids are just like her—'cept we got three of them."

Years go by and your daughter has yet to intellectualize danger, fear, gravity, pain. At Costco you've lost her twice. There are terrifying seconds after you realize she is gone, gone! And she'd go off with anyone. Anyone holds out a hand, she would take it. But there she is at the video bins. . . . Later she puts her hand through a plate glass window. You don't notice until, filling the hummingbird feeder, you glance at her shredded arm. Waiting in the ER presents another nightmare, a treadmill of Kafkaesque absurdities. Like your kid is going to sit in a chair for three or four or five hours. Right. Must keep moving. So you walk with her without rest. Gliding together in sweeping, repetitive loops throughout the waiting room, holding her arm upward as much as possible. Still, she manages to lunge for strangers' drinks, hoot and scream inappropriately, bolt down hallways. She is atomic. She is the nucleus around which her positively charged parents rotate—or deflect from—in collision. Finally, the triage nurse buzzes you in. "Oh, autistic? You should have said something. I would have bumped you." Taking her vitals is akin to restraining a wild animal. Half a dozen nurses, two paramedics, and some beefy security guys must hold her down forty minutes before the knockout drops relax her. All this for eight stitches.

Occasionally, guardian angels materialize. A young woman who bonds with your child like some mysterious winged sibling. But eventually they must leave, to pursue a career in special education or guide rafters

in Wyoming. Departments of developmental disabilities, in their infinite
wisdom, offer alternatives under the auspices of placement vendors who
contract with lowest-bidder employment agencies. Minimum-wage high
school grads show up at your door, thick as a brick, snapping gum, caked
in makeup, don't know autism from order-of-fries-with-that? So you train
them. It's either that or quit your job so somebody is home after school.
Well, the new gal is finally enough along that you figure she can handle
taking her charge out in public. The cops explain later that your daughter
caused such a scene in the parking lot of Target somebody thought a kid-
napping was in progress. Her new aide, useless, tugging on the screaming
preteen, became hysterical when the police arrived. The sheriff's helicopter, whirling figure eights, exacerbates everything. Your daughter, you
are told, was unresponsive to police commands, resisted contact. She was
handcuffed after attempting to bite one of the officers.

In the apocalypse scenario, your nightmare—infrastructure cleaved, roads
clogged, ERs overwhelmed—your kid drags down the entire family. As
does the diabetic kid, the wheelchair kid. Does someone stay behind so
that the family may survive? Or does the family reject this, insisting the
unit stay whole while around them entropy multiplies?

From North America to Europe to Australia the infanticide news
items shadow your conscience. In Southern California, a father shoots
his twenty-seven-year-old son to death and then himself. You must acknowledge that you know this man. You have seen him in your coffee,
the windshield, the mirror. A father approaching sixty. The young adult
under his roof knocking him down reaching for the cereal. A succession
of in-home aides quit. The mother, fighting her own infirmities, avoids
her son. Placement in group homes refused. Siblings say, "I got my own
problems." The father sees his son in ten years locked away somewhere.
Forgotten. No advocate. No family. No warmth of touch. Who will care
what his pleasures are? Will someone ever take him rafting down the Bit-
terroot again? The father sees his son wandering hallways the rest of his
life. Soiled pajamas. Decaying teeth. His only human contact a brusque
toweling down after a lukewarm shower.

For most people, autism, like abstract art or Alzheimer's or astrophysics, remains startling and unfathomable. For parents, the raising of children with severe disabilities confirms the indifference of nature, the disorder of the universe. Any potential, any ambition they once may have entertained for themselves has forever been compromised. Together with their remarkable, impossible children they make a life on a different planet. Where the gravity is very strong. And the climate rarely changes.

the day the world split open

ABIGAIL THOMAS

My husband and I met twelve years ago after he answered a personal ad I placed in the *New York Review of Books*. We met at the Moon Palace restaurant on Broadway and 112th Street. It was raining; he carried a big umbrella. He had beef with scallions, and I had sliced sautéed fish. It took me about five minutes to realize this was the nicest man in the world; and when he asked me to marry him thirteen days later, I said yes. He was fifty-seven, I was forty-six. Why wait?

We still have the magazine. I used to look at the page full of ads, mine the only one he'd circled, and feel the fragility of our luck. "Thank you for the happiest year of my life," he wrote on our first anniversary. We envisioned an old age on a front porch somewhere, each other's comfort, companions for life. But life takes twists and turns. There is good luck and bad.

Yesterday in his hospital room my husband asked urgently, "Will you move me 26,000 miles to the left?" "Yes," I said, not moving from my chair. After a moment he said, "Thank you," adding in wonder, "I didn't feel a thing." "You're welcome," I answered. "Are we alone?" he asked. "We are," I answered, the nurse's aide having stepped out for a moment. "What happened to Stacy and the flounder?" he said, and I saw the hospital room as he must experience it, a kind of primordial twilight soup, an atmosphere in which a flounder might well be swimming through midair. The image stays with me.

My husband is having brain surgery next week, and I am sitting in the dog park. The weather is what Rich would call "a soft day." This is the place I try to make sense of things, order them, to tame what happened.

Our beagle, Harry, makes his way around the perimeter of the dog run with his nose to the ground. He is a loner. I, too, sit by myself, but I pay attention to everything. "Suffering is the finest teacher," said an old friend long ago. "It teaches you details." I didn't know what he was talking about. I do now. I watch the dogs, one tiny dachshund so skinny he looks like a single stroke of calligraphy. An elderly man with a very young chow reaches down to pat my dog. Harry skips away. "Very good," answers an- other man who has just been asked how he is. It has been a long time since I answered that question that way.

Monday, April 24, at nine-forty at night, our doorman Pedro called me on the intercom. "Your dog is in the elevator," he said. The world had just changed forever, and I think I knew it even then. "My dog? Where is my husband?" I asked. "I don't know. But your dog is in the elevator with 14E, you better go get him." I stepped into the hall in my bathrobe. The elevator door opened, and a neighbor delivered Harry to me. "Where is my husband?" I asked again, but my neighbor didn't know. Harry was trembling. Rich must be frantic, I thought. Then the buzzer rang again. "Your husband has been hit by a car," Pedro said, "Riverside and 113th. Hurry."

Impossible, impossible. Where were my shoes? My skirt? I was in slow motion, moving underwater. I looked under the bed, found my left shoe, grabbed a sweater off the back of a chair. This couldn't be serious. I threw my clothes on and got into the elevator. Then I ran along Riverside, and when I saw the people on the sidewalk ahead I began to run faster, calling his name. What kind of injury drew such a crowd?

I found my husband lying in the middle of a pool of blood, his head split open. Red lights were flashing from cop cars and emergency vehicles, and the EMS people were kneeling over his body. "Let them work," said a police officer as I tried to fight my way next to him, managing to get close enough to touch his hand. They were cutting the clothes off him, his windbreaker, his flannel shirt. Somebody pulled me away. "Don't look," he said, but I needed to look, I needed to keep my eyes on him. A police- man began asking me questions. "You're his wife? What's his name? Date of birth? What's your name? Address?" Then, as I watched, they loaded Rich onto a stretcher and into the ambulance. I wanted to climb in, too, but they sped off without me. A policeman drove me to the emergency room at St. Luke's Hospital, three blocks away. The superintendent of our building, Cranston Scott, came with me, stayed until my family arrived, gave me his credit card number to call my children and my sisters. I called Rich's former wife, who had the numbers of Rich's children, his brother Gil. I waited in a small room outside the emergency room at the hospital while dozens of hospital personnel went through the door where my husband lay. I found out later that the accident report the police filled out listed Rich as "dead, or likely to die."

Harry wanders over. He looks up at me, and I reach down to stroke his head, his ears. He comes to me to reassure himself that I am still there, I think, or perhaps to reassure me that he is still there. He was a stray; we adopted him from a friend into whose yard he had wandered, starved and terrified, a year ago. Rich hadn't wanted a dog. Every time I dragged him to look at yet another puppy I'd discovered in yet another pet store, he would look at it and say something like, "Yes, but isn't his face a bit rodentlike?" When I took him to meet Harry he said, "Well, that's a very nice little dog." Five months later, Harry got off his leash and Rich ran into Riverside Drive to save him. I don't look at Harry and think, *If only we hadn't got him.* I don't blame myself for this accident, or our dog, although I believe if it had been a child who was hurt, I probably would. We were two adults living our lives, and this terrible thing happened. I don't find it ironic that the very reason Rich got hurt is the creature who comforts me. There is no irony here, no room for guilt or second-guessing. That would be a diversion, an indulgence. These are hard facts to be faced head-on. We are in this together, my husband and I, we have been thrown into this unfamiliar country with different weather, different rules. Everything I think and do matters now, in a way it never has before.

I seem to be leaving in the road behind me all sorts of unnecessary baggage, stuff too heavy to carry. Old fears are evaporating: the claustrophobia that crippled me for years is gone, vanished. I used to climb the thirteen flights to our apartment because I was terrified of being alone in the elevator. What if it got stuck? What if I never got out? Then there I was one Sunday morning in the hospital, Rich on the eighth floor, the elevator empty. What had for years terrified me now seemed ridiculously easy. I haven't got the time for this, I thought, and got right in. When the doors closed, I kept thinking, *Go ahead! Try it! What more can you possibly do to me?*

The head injury my husband sustained is a traumatic brain injury, specifically damage to the frontal lobes; part of his brain has descended into his sinus cavities, dragging arteries along with it. There is a hole or holes in his dura, the casing around the brain; his skull is fractured like a spider web. Everywhere. The danger of meningitis is real. They must remove the dead brain tissue, repair the dura, relieve the pressure in the buildup of fluid, repair the damage to his skull. It is a long surgery and carries with it its own danger of infection. The surgery was scheduled three weeks ago, but had to be postponed when Rich developed a fever three days before.

He was fine in the morning and in a good mood, but by afternoon he felt warm to my touch, and he was unlike himself, unlike any version of himself. He spoke in a low, raspy voice like Jimmy Cagney, and I couldn't reel him back from the deep water he seemed to be in. I knew that one of the early signs of meningitis is a personality change, and I was scared. The doctors immediately treated him as if this were meningitis, and bags of sinister yellow liquids dripped into his arm. The lumbar puncture came back negative, but the surgery was postponed until his fever went down.

It is June, the weather is warm, and Harry is shedding. When I brush him he stands absolutely still. At night he sleeps in bed with me. I feel his warm breath on my neck, his ear "like a velvet lily pad," as Rich described it, against my cheek. I don't sleep on Rich's side of the bed, Rich's side is Rich's side, his pajamas still neatly tucked under his pillow. When I first saw them, and his trousers over the back of the chair, I wept. When I think about the past I get sad, our mornings of coffee and the newspaper. Rich looking out the window at any kind of weather, sun, pouring rain, and saying, "Good day for a run." He was a runner, fast and full of endurance, and when we got married I made him put his trophies on our wall. After his shower he would appear in the kitchen with the bathroom wastebasket in his hands, announcing "the naked dustman." I miss my husband. I miss the comfort of living with this man I loved and trusted absolutely. When I gave a reading in May, I missed his shining face among the others.

I missed his pride in me, his impulse to take everyone in the audience out for dinner. Walking down our street, I missed him by my side. The past gets swallowed up in the extraordinary circumstances of now. But mostly it hurts too much to let my mind go back.

My son called last night. "Are you worried about the operation?" he asked. "I don't think so," I answered. It is what I have heard one of the surgeons call "meat and potatoes surgery." What terrifies me is seeing Rich in the recovery room. This doesn't make any sense, but I keep remembering his face just after his accident, ruined beyond recognition, blood pooling in the corners of his swollen eyes. Those first days his daughter Sally and I took twelve-hour shifts at the hospital, sitting in a chair next to his bed, listening to the beeping of monitors in the ICU. We were afraid to leave him. It was as if we were trying to hatch an egg, keeping him warm with our presence, and we didn't want him to wake without a familiar face nearby. "Que pasa?" were the first words he spoke when the doctors removed his breathing tube. I put my ear close to his mouth. "Que pasa?" This man who failed Spanish. It is a funny miracle.

I am sitting on my bench; behind me, three dogs are digging a hole to China. The odd woman who wears a bandage across her nose and white gloves, who often stands at the gate excoriating dogs and their owners with tales of being trailed by the FBI, has just sat down next to me. She has a whippet. Whippets, she tells me, were dogs that hunted rats in the mines. "Wales, or Scotland or Ireland," she goes on. There being no room to break their necks in the small spaces they twirled and twirled, snapping the rat's necks that way. "That's interesting," I say cautiously. Talk moves on and about, like a dog looking for a good place to lie down. Somehow we speak of the old radio shows. *Clyde Beatty, Sky King, Sergeant Preston of the Yukon.* She asks do I remember the real-estate offering they made? I shake my head. "You could buy one inch in Alaska," she says. All day I can't get the idea of owning an inch of the Alaskan wilderness out of my head. I am searching for meaning in everything.

In the first weeks after his accident, Rich spoke in mysteries. It was as if he were now connected to some vast reservoir of wisdom, available only to those whose brains have been altered, a reservoir unencumbered by personality, quirks, history, habits. "It is interesting to think that one could run further and longer and perhaps find the answer," he said one evening, drifting in and out of delirious talk. "What would you get to?" I asked, eager for the answer. "The allure of distance," was what he said, a dreamy phrase. Last week, as he struggled to make sense of the world, unable to find words, my daughter Catherine came to visit. "Do you know who I am?" she asked. He peered at her intently. "Do you eat field mice?" he asked, a strange question, we thought, until I realized the first three letters of her name spell "cat." Perhaps this was a glimpse of how the mind pieces things together after an assault, trying to rewire itself. "The goat's mouth is full of stones," he said one day, and I leave that as it is, a mystery. During the days when it is impossible to communicate in words, I get into his bed and we hold hands. Nap therapy. This is a familiar posture, something we can do without speech, without thinking.

"How are you managing?" friends ask. "How are you doing this?" They leave me food and flowers; they send me letters and messages. They pray. I love these people, I love my family. Doing what? I wonder. This is the path our lives have taken. A month ago I would have thought this life impossible. Sometimes I feel as if I'm trying to rescue a drowning man, and I only have time to rise to the surface for one gasp of air before I go back down again. There is an exhilaration to it, a high born only partly of exhaustion, and I find myself almost frighteningly alive. There is nothing like calamity for refreshing the moment. Ironically, the last several years my life had begun to feel shapeless, like underwear with the elastic gone, the days down around my ankles. Now there is an intensity to the humblest things—buying paper towels, laundry detergent, dog food, keeping the household running in Rich's absence. One morning I buy myself a necklace made of sea glass, and it becomes a talisman. Shopping contains the future. As my daughter Jennifer says, shopping is hope.

On the day of Rich's surgery, his daughter Sally and I are there at 6:30 in the morning to accompany him to the operating room. We walk beside the stretcher and try to calm him, but he is disoriented and very agitated, until the anesthesiologist starts the Demerol drip. "Can we get some of that to go?" asks Sally. When they wheel him into the operating theater, we go to have breakfast in the hospital cafeteria. Sally has two boiled eggs, Cream of Wheat, corned beef hash, and coffee. She's a nurse, and she

knows what she's doing: it's going to be a long day. I have a banana. The
waiting room is a large place with high ceilings, and through a sliver of
window I can see the brightly colored clothes of pint-size campers out on
Fifth Avenue with their nannies, the green of Central Park behind them.
Outside the weather is cool and clear, and Sally and I settle down for the
long wait. The surgery is expected to take all day. I am not worried about
Rich, but my dog has gotten sick: his ears were hot and he didn't eat; his
stool was bloody. My sister has agreed to take him to the vet. Suddenly
panicky, I begin calling my sister every fifteen minutes. Patiently her son
tells me his mother is still at the vet. I can't think straight. What would I
do without Harry? Finally in my desperation I call the vet himself. It turns
out Harry has colitis, and all I need to do is feed him lots of rice and give
him medicine for five days. This is such a huge relief that I wonder for
a second why I was so worried, and then it hits me: I comfort Rich but
Harry comforts me.

At six o'clock we find out that Rich's surgery has gone well. We can
go up and see him in the recovery room, the SICU. He is asleep, bandages
around his head; beneath them are the staples that cross his head from ear
to ear. The doctors have done what they set out to do. There being no bone
left unsplintered in his forehead (shattered like an eggshell, they tell us), they
have built him a new one, made of titanium. They have rebuilt the floor of
his brain; they have removed the dead tissue. The brain fluid that had been
building up is relieved. His right frontal lobe is gone, and the left damaged.
They tell us again that there will be differences in Rich's personality and
that only time will tell the nature of the changes. I have never processed
this information. Changes? Just give him back to me and everything will
be all right. We begin the round of phone calls to friends and family.

But in the days immediately following the surgery Rich enters the
stage known as "inappropriate behavior." This is a euphemism for the anger and irrationality that is part of the process of recovery. Rich is angry
and confused. He doesn't mention going home; there is no destination
except "out of here." I betray him all the time, he says, by not saving him.
He thought he could trust me, he thought we loved each other, but now
our love seems very thin to him, he says. Roughly, he pushes my hand
away as I reach for his. My feelings are hurt—I can't help it—although I

try to reason them away. Sitting with him hour after hour, his face glowering, makes me think of the stories I've heard of people who after traumatic brain injury bore no resemblance to their former selves. I am terrified that a change like this will undo me. This man is not the man I married. None of this is his doing—he didn't choose this; but neither did I.

One day I look out the hospital window high above Central Park, and I feel as if there's a tightrope connecting Rich's hospital room to our apartment, and all I do is walk back and forth on it, the city far below. I can almost see it shivering like a high-tension wire above the trees. This is when I learn that I have to take care of myself, even if my leaving makes him angry, or worse, sad. I need to eat and sleep. I need to do something mindless, go to a movie, fritter away an afternoon. And I realize something even more startling: I can't make everything all right. It's his body that is hurt, not mine. I can't fix it, I can't make it never have happened.

Rich still refuses food and medicine; everything has been poisoned. "Why are you so fatuous?" he asks angrily as I try to say something cheery about the potassium in a banana. Remarks like this sting me, especially because I sound like Pollyanna even to myself. When we wheel him down a hospital hall for a CAT scan, he says, "You always know you're in for it when you're going down a long hall with nobody else in it." Afterward he tells me, "I felt I was at a casual execution." When he's lost almost thirty pounds, they put a peg in his stomach. Through this tube, which resembles a monkey's tail as it curls out from under the covers to the IV pole, they give him nourishment and medicine. The shape of the tube may be what gives rise to Rich's belief that there is literally a monkey in the bed. "There's no monkey," I tell him. "Don't be so sure," he says, lifting the sheet to peer beneath it.

How do I separate the old Rich from this new Rich—what allowances do I make for his injury, when do I draw the line? How do I draw the line? The nurses say this is just a stage, but I can't seem to sweep it under the rug. I can't even locate the rug. I miss my old husband. I miss the old me. When I run across something from before the accident, a snapshot of Rich smiling his beautiful smile, I feel such staggering loss. What happened? Where did my husband go? I clean the closet and find a tiny portable fan Rich bought me for trips because I can't sleep without white noise, and it makes me cry.

"I don't know who I am," Rich says over and over. "There are too many thoughts inside my head. I am not myself." Yesterday he said, "Pretend you are walking up the street with your friend. You are looking in windows. But right behind you is a man with a huge roller filled with white paint and he is painting over everywhere you've been, erasing everything. He erases your friend. You don't even remember his name." The image makes me shiver, but he seems exultant in his description. There are days when he is grounded in the here and now and days when his brain is boiling over with confusion. When he is angry, I go home after only a short visit. Staying does neither of us any good. Where do I put these bad days? Part of me is still hanging on to the couple we were. Where do I put my anger? What right have I to be angry? My husband is hurt. Part of him is destroyed. I don't even feel my anger most of the time, but it's there, and I only acknowledge it when I find myself doing something self-destructive—going for a day or two without eating, drinking too much coffee, allowing myself to get lonely, tired.

"Good things happen slowly," said a doctor in the ICU months ago, "and bad things happen fast." Those were comforting words, and they comfort me today. Recovery is a long, slow process. There are good days and bad days for both of us. I try to find an even keel, but still I am upset on the bad days and hopeful on the good. Uncertainty is the hardest part. There is no prognosis; no one can tell me how much better Rich will get and how long it might take. The day before my birthday, Rich imagines that we've gone to Coney Island and that he bought me a shell necklace. This is my present, as real for me as it was for him. He held my hand. That was yesterday, a good day, but filled with sadness. The season is changing. I take Harry to the park and watch the leaves turning and falling; there is beauty overhead and underfoot. There is something else I don't know yet, something I'm straining to feel, as subtle as the change in humidity or temperature, or the shift in light as summer becomes fall, the most beautiful season, with its gift of beauty in loss, and the promise of something more to come.

the elephant in the room

This is the story of a love affair.

For eighteen years Janet Bode and I lived, worked and traveled together. We were almost never apart. And we never married. She'd say, "Why fix it if it ain't broke?" And I enjoyed that little thrill of the illicit.

I wonder now whether, even if we had chosen marriage, I would have thought any more deeply about the implications of the marriage vows "In sickness and in health, till death do us part." Who thinks about sickness and death when you're starting a life together?

Janet was fun and exciting; we were healthy and in love, and that was plenty. We focused on our work—she as a writer of nonfiction books for teenagers, I as a cartoonist. The future would take care of itself.

In those early days, I could never have imagined how much our relationship would transform my thinking about what was important in life, and what love is.

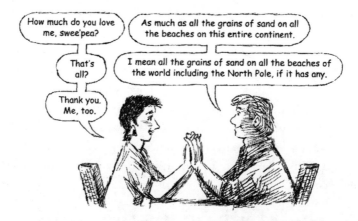

Little by little, as the years went by, and without at first realizing it, Janet and I built bridges to each other that would sustain us during the coming tough times.

In 1994 Janet was diagnosed with breast cancer. Her offbeat spirit and humor carried us through a year of treatment and three years of remission. The cancer returned in the fall of 1998.

Through the time of her illness, I learned to be both tender and strong. And when, as her condition worsened, I weakened, I also found I could recover. I now believe that a loving partner can help you find strengths within yourself that you didn't know were there.

When things got really bad, Janet continued to give me the trust that allowed me to help her; she even, I felt, showed me the way. Though I'd never taken care of a sick person and had never heard the term *primary caregiver*, that's what I did and that's what I became.

Janet stood up to her cancer and continued to embrace life. She fiercely held on to her belief in her own value—she refused to fade into neutral. She lost her temper, gossiped with friends, and made (sometimes bad) jokes about her disease. She never succumbed to despair. And she never stopped loving me.

Now I understand that the end is always part of the beginning. For every one of us, there will come a time of parting . . . and an afterwards. Janet lived for her season. Then, like a runner in a relay race, she passed on her love of life to me.

On December 30, 1999, at about 6:30 A.M., one day before the end of the millennium, she died. Thankfully, it was in our home, our little loft in Greenwich Village, New York City. She was fifty-six years old.

• • •

Throughout her treatment, Janet believed she was getting the best medicine available—though she was not naïve about the capabilities of the

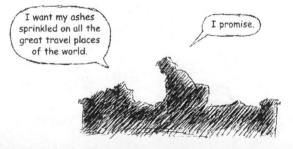

> I want my ashes sprinkled on all the great travel places of the world.

> I promise.

doctors. She was open to the alternative remedies, far-out offerings, good luck charms, protective totems, and spiritual amulets contributed by her friends. But the best medicine arrived in the early summer of 1999 from an unexpected source. The editor of *Natural History* magazine asked me to do a humorous piece on the solar eclipse that August—during a special eclipse cruise leaving from Greece and sailing the Black Sea. This was the kind of assignment Janet and I dreamed of. My first thought was of Janet. How could I go without her, yet how could she go? Janet took care of that question right away and immediately began the planning that would keep her engaged for the next two months.

Janet became so busy with our plans for the Black Sea voyage on a ship (that now included NASA scientists and two former astronauts)—she didn't have room in her day for thoughts of dying.

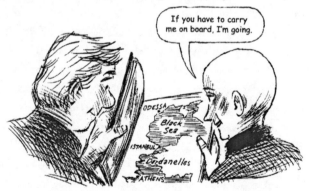

Janet and I met Carolyn and Mike, Kathryn and Larry in Athens, and we boarded the ship. We sailed for the Black Sea, stopping at the Temple of Asclepius (the Greek god of healing), the Blue Mosque in Istanbul, the

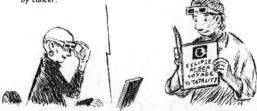

Getting ready for our trip to the Black Sea. Yippee! Sister Carolyn with boyfriend Mike and friend Kathryn with boyfriend Larry have decided to join us. We'll rendezvous in Athens. The New York Times said the region is dangerous for travel right now. I say better to die on an adventure than incrementally by cancer.

Potemkin Steps in Odessa. Janet, using a cane and moving slowly, came ashore every time.

On the day of the eclipse, while I worked on my assignment, our friends carried Janet in a wheelchair up an outside ladder to the observation deck for a front-row seat of the spectacle. She wore a wide-brimmed hat, long scarf, single hoop earring, and dark glasses. She looked mysterious and beautiful.

We arrived home on Friday, August 13. In an e-mail a few days later, she described the experience.

But she came home with a raging fever and in hellish pain.

Janet's doctor, Laura, evaluated Janet's condition and told us that the current chemo wasn't working well enough to continue. We now under-

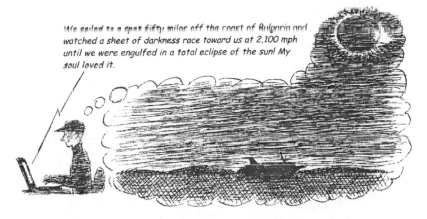

We sailed to a spot fifty miles off the coast of Bulgaria and watched a sheet of darkness race toward us at 2,100 mph until we were engulfed in a total eclipse of the sun! My soul loved it.

stood that it was the cancer itself, rather than the chemo, that was causing much of her pain.

But Laura told us there were still treatment options. She put Janet on a second chemo drug, Navelbine, and brought in a pain specialist, who recommended methadone. It turned out to be far more effective in combating Janet's pain than the morphine she'd been taking.

Laura's discussions with Janet about treatment side effects like nausea, pain, and even about alternative remedies were straightforward and helpful. Janet said their conversations were good therapy. However, Laura's approach to the true course of Janet's disease remained ambiguous.

Janet's fate was like the proverbial invisible elephant living in our apartment. Something was crashing around and hurting us both, but we didn't know what. We needed someone to talk honestly, not just about the

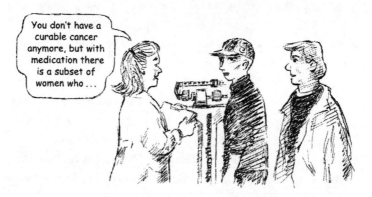

details of coping with neuropathy, constipation, and bone pain, but about the !@#$%! elephant.

How much improvement could we expect from the new chemo? What physiological changes should we prepare for, and how should we handle them? Was she terminal? If so, how much time did she have? Who

was to tell us what we didn't know to ask?

One day in September, Janet and I were on the street, and she noticed a few early dead leaves on the sidewalk. "Oh dear," she lamented, "fall is here!" We used to joke about how Janet always hated fall. To me, it was a time of brilliant colors and welcome coolness. To her, it was a gloomy herald of winter's doom. That fall Janet's health would slide inexorably down.

Up till now, Janet was in charge of her illness. I was her chief cook, bottle washer, and faithful backup. Now as pain and treatment wore her down, she needed me to step out in front and take on more of the medical decision making.

She had pills for pain, spiking pain, strength, nausea, bowel movements, tingling of fingers and toes. . . . I would wake up in the middle of the night to see her, woozy from drugs, gripping her pen and yellow legal pad, struggling to keep track of the symptoms and medications. And I knew it was only going to get worse.

I urged her to get one of those weekly pill organizers. At first she resisted; she'd always relied on her yellow legal pad. Finally she agreed. I took over the job of organizing the pills and made sure she took the right

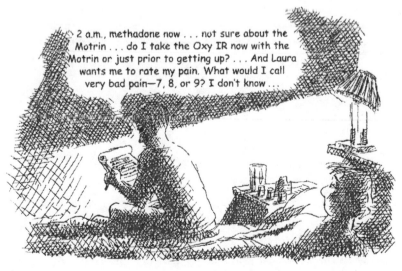

ones at the right time, day and night. It was important to both of us that she was the one to make the decision to delegate the job to me.

We were now entering a darker world of ever more disheartening medical problems. Janet began to lose bladder control—a situation we tried to make light of.

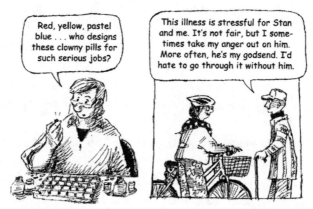

I knew there were handheld plastic urinals that she could keep by the bed at night. I found my way to Bigelow's medical supply store, not far from our apartment. I bought a female urinal and a rubber sheet and came

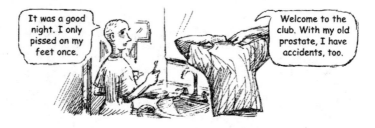

back in triumph. Problem solved.

But the problems never stayed solved. They only got worse.

Janet's nightly incidents increased. I went back to Bigelow's and bought a plastic bedpan. This time I walked the aisles, reading labels on adult diapers, bathroom grab bars, shower seats, walkers, sipping cups . . . giving myself a crash course on what might lie ahead.

Eventually we switched from the bedpan to a full-sized bedside commode. I remember walking home on a sunny Saturday afternoon with the commode in my arms, passing strolling couples. I imagined them making cracks to each other about the guy with the toilet.

One day I returned from Bigelow's proud of the good deal I got on a four-footed cane. But soon Janet felt more secure with the extra stability of a walker. Then a wheelchair. Janet joked about doing wheelies while

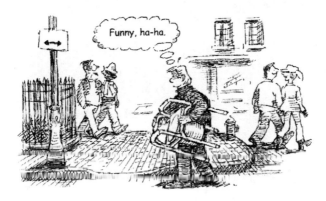

the canes and walker stood in the corners of the apartment, silent reminders of just last week.

With the wheelchair, the five steps in front of our building, which had been nearly invisible to us before, loomed like Everest. I could look for help each time but, practically, we were trapped. I researched city

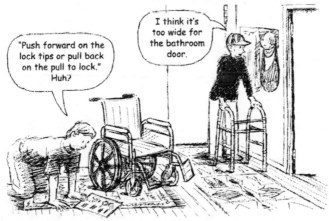

regulations, went online, talked to the building's management. I believed that if I found the right ramp for our sidewalk and door, Janet would be free again.

But it didn't really matter. Once in the wheelchair, she went out less and less.

All this time, Janet had been going to the hospital for chemo, scans, and blood transfusions. The doctors and technicians cared not at all how we got to them as long as we showed up on time. The cost, the pain, the

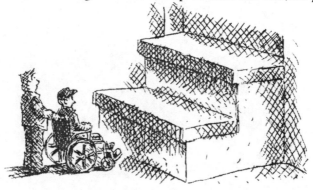

logistics—all ours. As Janet became less mobile, our transportation changed from bus to cab; once we even hired an ambulance. But we mostly used ambulettes, whose drivers varied from caring to dangerous.

Ambulette: van that transports patients who can sit up. It can securely carry wheelchairs. Driver and helper are not required to have any medical training.

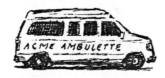

Ambulance: vehicle that transports bed-confined patients by stretcher. Driver and helper are both emergency medical technicians. The vehicle is outfitted with emergency equipment.

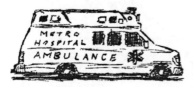

Jeannie, a friend from Seattle, came to visit Janet late in October. She went with Janet to one of her blood transfusions. I hadn't had any sleep the night before and needed a nap. Jeannie remembered a harrowing ride home.

"Janet threw up while we waited for the ambulette, which arrived late. The driver was hostile, didn't strap the wheelchair down securely, and had his girlfriend with him. Janet gave him directions, trying to be friendly. Meanwhile, he's a motor mouth and she's bouncing around because of his careless driving.

"Janet realizes he's not taking us straight home, and she has to go to the bathroom. Janet's sleepy with painkillers, and she's fearful of breaking bones. I'm now convinced the driver is on speed.

"He finally drops off his girlfriend downtown. Suddenly, Janet wakes up and starts letting him have it. I'm yelling at him, too. And *he's* yelling about regulations.

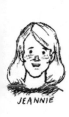

JEANNIE

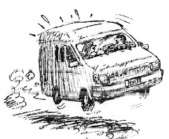

"We make it to the apartment and Janet is swearing about the driver and even grumbling at Stan. I was thinking, Sixty dollars for *that?* This is what it's like being sick in New York?"

Even hospitals, supposedly centers of safety and healing, could be hazardous to your health. One day in October, Janet woke up with extreme hip pain. Laura had her admitted to the hospital for observation. In Janet's room, the patient in the adjoining bed was lying in her own waste and appeared to be moaning for help. At the end of visiting hours, they told me I had to leave. I should have insisted on staying, but I left at 11:00 P.M., planning to be back first thing in the morning. Janet called me in the middle of the night, crying. "I'm on the cuckoo's nest floor. The nurses and attendants are mean, sloppy, and uncaring."

I rushed over early in the morning to find her distraught.

In the corridor, I ran into Danny, an intern we'd met during an earlier hospital stay. He used his clout to get Janet released quickly.

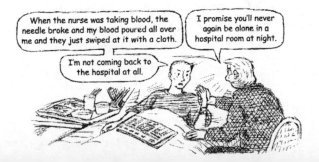

Later Laura said, "Oh yes, that's a bad floor, but it was the only bed available."

As we were waiting to leave, I told Danny we really needed help at home. He walked us to a door that said "Social Worker."

The social worker rushed in, listened to our story, and signed us up with a CHHA (certified home health agency). The social worker said they provide various skilled home services, and she rushed off again—another patient successfully released.

So there actually was a system in place. We just didn't know what it was.

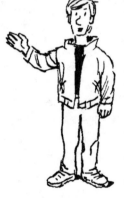

The Way It Works: If the patient requires more nursing help than you can provide, your doctor can authorize home care. The doctor or hospital will contact a CHHA on your behalf. The CHHA will work with your insurance carrier to see how many—or how few—visits your plan covers. The CHHA will assign a visiting nurse to your case. The nurse, in consultation with your doctor, will evaluate your needs and can request such additional services as a visiting physical therapist and home health-care aide and equipment such as a commode and wheelchair.

It looked like we would finally have skilled help—though I didn't even know the difference between a nurse and a home health-care aide.

Visiting Nurses: Visiting nurses are directed by the doctor. They evaluate, take vital signs, give medication and injections, and do postsurgery follow-up. The visits are usually brief.

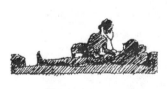

Home Health-Care Aides: Aides do basic health tasks related to the patient such as changing diapers and bedclothes, assisting in feeding and bathing, and doing laundry and errands. They are employed to stay with the patient.

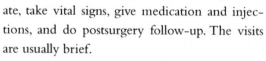

We were contacted by a caseworker, who assigned us a nurse, a social worker, a physical therapist, and a home health-care aide. The nurse visited twice a week. We were one of many on his route; he was almost like a paperboy the way he ran around the neighborhood. He took Janet's vital signs but was not permitted to answer our medical questions.

The social worker arrived and chatted for an hour—mostly about his upcoming retirement.

The physical therapist came weekly. He seemed better suited to working with football players, complained about his own bad back, and left Janet in worse pain.

When the home health aide appeared, we were excited—we would

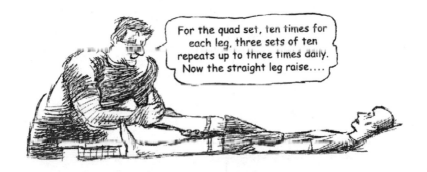

finally be getting real, practical help. But she was very young, had never worked as an aide before, and didn't seem particularly interested in the job. She began by telling us what she wouldn't do. I fumed, then thanked her for coming and said we wouldn't be needing her services. She refused to leave. Finally our friend Linda took her by the hand and walked her out of the building.

By phone, I was lectured by the agency for not understanding how the system worked. Apparently I did not have the authority to dismiss the aide, because all decisions were being made by the CHHA and Janet's insurance company. Though it seems obvious now, we didn't realize then that we could go outside the system, hiring and paying for our own care. Janet and I made decisions based on the information we had.

Janet was eating less, and her tastes were changing. First she craved

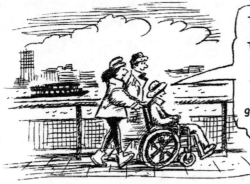

comfort foods like macaroni and cheese. Then she turned to soups and puddings, and then yogurt, health drinks, and fruit drinks. As she consumed less, I became a Jewish mother.

One day in October, a scary thought hit me: maybe she was trying to

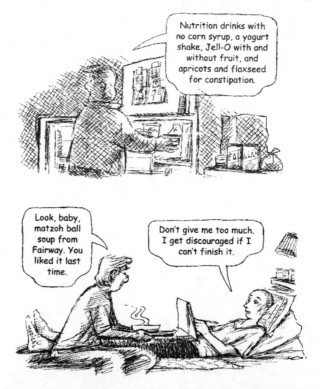

starve herself to death. I sat on the side of the bed and struggled to come out with the question. She looked at me with genuine surprise and said no. I realized she could never do such a life-denying thing and suddenly I was bawling—something I'd never done before in my life.

She didn't say anything, but the expression on her face made me wonder if she felt she now had to protect me.

Late in November our friend Kate came for a visit.

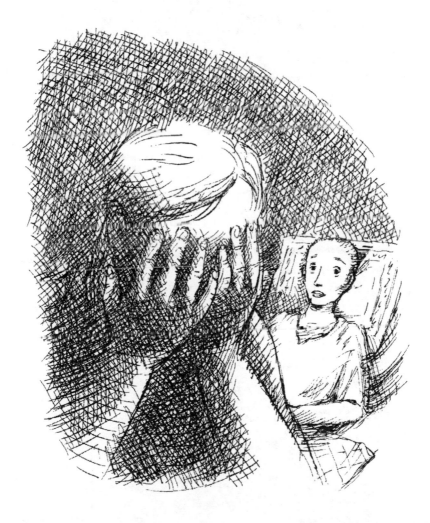

"The drugs were beginning to make Janet anxious. When she would become nervous, Stan would say:

"... and she would calm down. She was best when

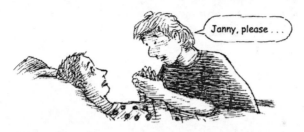

Janny, please . . .

he was near. There was a deliberate openness between them. My sense was she was also taking care of him.

"When I was rubbing her, she said to me: 'It was good with Stan, I love him, I am fortunate to have him. I have friends who care, I am at peace, I've had a good life.'

"Their apartment was a remarkably dignified place. When people arrived, Stan would orient them, bring them up to his level of caring. A visitor once said she's dying, and he got very angry. That was exactly not the point.

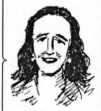

KATE

"I was worried that it was getting too much for Stan. I walked him to the river and said, 'You're getting depleted, you have no network of help. People on drugs can die suddenly and you won't be prepared.' I suggested hospice. He was afraid I was saying that he was supposed to have end-of-life conversations, and he laughed nervously."

Even when friends were helping, it was difficult hav-

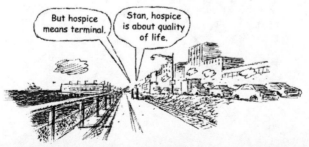

But hospice means terminal.

Stan, hospice is about quality of life.

ing visitors all the time. Janet would say, "We're tired. I love my dear friends, but Stan and I need to have our private time." The door would finally close on the last visitor, and we'd be alone.

In the quiet of those moments, Janet and I would reach out to each

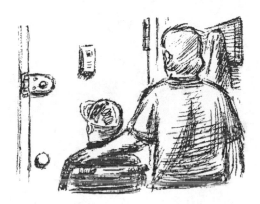

other and try to reconnect, try to feel ordinary again—talking about her twenty-pound weight loss that month and her urine-soaked towel the way we used to discuss publishers' contracts or the occasional mouse in the apartment.

We'd lie in bed watching reruns of *Law and Order* and *ER*—familiar

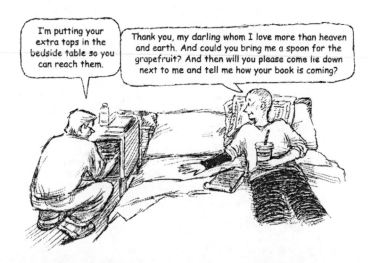

was good. Or we'd talk about nothing.

And sometimes she'd fall asleep, and I'd keep talking.

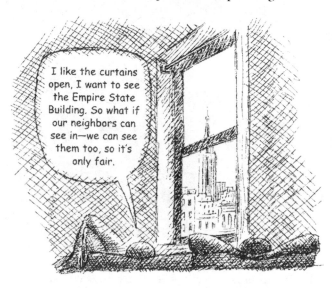

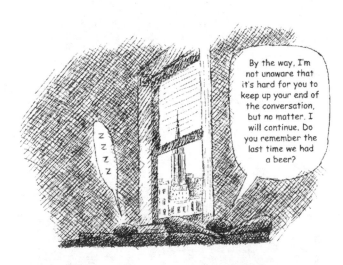

transformed by a touch

KERREL MCKAY

I was nine years old when I found out my father was ill. I can remember my mother's words, spoken in her rich Jamaican accent, as if it happened yesterday: "Kerrel, I don't want you to take food from your father, because him have the AIDS. Be very careful when you are around him."

I had not known that Daddy was ill. He visited me regularly—after my parents split up, I lived with my mother—and he was always energetic and attentive. I remember he would often take the biggest piece of chicken from his plate and hand it to me, even when I was too full to eat it. Even when he wasn't certain there'd be another meal like that soon again. I remember he used to take me on the porch of his house; we'd look out on the giant ackee tree in his yard, bursting with its luscious red fruits, and he'd ask me to spell *Catadupa*. This was his favorite word—it is the name of the town where he was from in Saint James Parish, Jamaica—and he'd always praise me after I'd say it, proud that his little girl could spell such a difficult word, and then he'd repeat the word himself, appreciating its melody. I remember he always laughed like there was no tomorrow at his own jokes, his head thrown back from his sturdy body in appreciation. Daddy was so life-giving, it was hard for me to imagine his own would ever be taken away.

My father's seeming good health, and my tender youth, were not the only reasons for my naïveté about his illness: We lived in Portland Parish, a rural part of Jamaica, on the northeast coast, where people knew so little of HIV/AIDS in 1993, the year my mother told me of my father's illness. Most people had not yet learned the facts about how the disease is contracted or how to prevent it from happening. There was still a mythical sense that the illness was simply hovering in the atmosphere, slyly waiting to find its way into the next person's body and life. AIDS was a forbidden word, the unspeakable, and no one wanted to be associated with it, including me. What we knew could be summed up like this: If you were HIV-positive, you were going to die. You were going to suffer before you died. And you couldn't expect anyone to treat you well, either. *Don't touch them, don't go near them, don't eat from them*: those were the warnings that went along with an AIDS patient in those days.

When my mother told me about my father's illness, she told me in a hushed and hurried whisper, setting the tone for how we'd handle it from then on. My father's illness was to be a secret. My mother asked me not to tell anyone, not even to let my father know that I knew. (After she was contacted for testing by the health department, my mother learned my father had HIV. Back then, the health department alerted the partners of the person who tested positive, without revealing the name of the patient. But my mother's one and only romance had been with Daddy. Daddy, on the other hand, had thirteen kids by four or five different women.) I understood—I *still* understand—why my mother didn't want people outside of our family to know about this. The stigma was too great; everyone would have treated us differently. I had seen kids taunted and teased by classmates about parents with AIDS. Even adults could be cruel. We would have all suffered from the ridicule and alienation. But I wanted, *needed* more than anything, to talk about the circumstances with someone. It cost me more than any one of us could have imagined to keep this story inside for as long as I did.

For the first three years, though, Daddy seemed so much the same man to me, I sometimes forgot he was sick. There was nothing physically different about him. When I looked at him, I saw Daddy, and he looked just like me, so I didn't see anything that I should fear. And he was still able to be a father to me: He always made sure that I had lunch money and school supplies. If I had a complaint about anything, I could go to him and he would make sure to do something about it. I visited him every Sunday. He would tell me how grateful he was, how glad he was that I was there. But the conversation never went further. I always thought he would one day finally say *it,* and we would talk about what was happening, that he was living with HIV.

By the time I was twelve, my father had succumbed to the illness much more visibly. My older siblings were living elsewhere—nearly half of them had moved to the United States—and the only way that they could contribute was to send a little money when Daddy needed it. (Later, I would discover that not even my sisters and brothers knew Daddy had AIDS. They simply knew he was very ill.) It became clear that my father needed help, and it fell to me to look after him. I tended to his every need. After school, I would cook, clean, shop for groceries, and take Daddy to the doctor. His cries and complaints from chronic headaches became the norm, and rubbing cream over his itching and aching body was something I would fast learn to do. Doing his laundry, cleaning the house, and making his breakfast also found its place during my visits. Daddy tried to be normal, to do some of the regular things we used to do, but I could see how much effort this took. Sometimes he would surrender to his emotions and say, "I'm going to die." I would cry every time I heard those words, but still there was never an explanation behind them. And because I was young and afraid and wishing it not to be true, I never asked anything further.

My mother both encouraged and feared the care I gave my father. She warned me often not to get infected, to do what I had to do to look after Daddy but to look out for myself, too. I remember once when I was doing the laundry, I found blood on my father's clothes. I let the water run really, really hard, until the blood ran out. From then on, I would touch his clothing but I would never touch the blood.

I stopped having any time for myself. My friends played at home during the summer, but I had to work. Somehow I had passed my exam for high school and maintained grades that kept me in the top ten of my class. I have no idea how I did that; in part I think it was my strong hope to elevate myself from the situation that I was living in. Still, I was struggling with depression, and each day brought with it a sense of gloom instead of hope.

Money was also a problem. We couldn't afford all the necessary medication for Daddy—he wasn't even taking medication for HIV (it wasn't available to him and, even if it had been, it would have been too expensive); he was being treated for his headaches and skin irritations—and he was getting weaker as a result. Since he was no longer able to do the work he'd once done at the wharf, I had no money for school supplies. Often, I couldn't even buy food for dinner. My mother was working as a chef at the time, but her income was not enough to pay bills, buy groceries, *and* send me to school. I borrowed pencils from classmates and shared textbooks. I took very good care of my uniform and shoes in order to preserve the little that we did have. Most of the time, I sat in class feeling completely lost, the teacher's words muffled as I tried to figure out how exactly I was going to manage.

I started to have nightmares, one terrifying dream right after the other. I can't remember the images now, I can only remember that when night came, I would start to sob because I was afraid to go to sleep. I begged my mother to stay up with me. She told me not to worry. She reminded me this would all be over soon. But that was what was haunting me: My father would soon be gone.

I was afraid of growing up without Daddy. He always made a big deal about my grades or any recognition I got in school. I wanted him to be a part of anything else I might achieve in life. I wanted to be his little girl. That child who never got the chance to grow still cries out in me; she is still longing to be released. My life was being devoured by Daddy's terrible fate, by these uninvited forces. I started thinking about how to end my own life in order not to have to face how I would suffer when Daddy lost his.

I did not share my burden with anyone. I did not talk to my parents about the pressure I was feeling. I did not talk to my friends about the fact that suicidal thoughts visited my mind often; that I had come to believe that being dead was a better option than living. I did not talk to anyone, because I was crippled by fear.

On the day that I gave up, when I was fifteen years old, I was cruelly punished. I told my mother that I was going to skip my visit with Daddy, I wanted to stay home and rest. She told me to make a very quick visit, but I refused. I called his neighbor instead. I was afraid if I called Daddy directly, he would be upset with me for not coming to see him. His neighbor said,

"I haven't seen your father since morning. The house has been locked up all day." Fear erupted throughout my body.

When I got to my father's house, I could see the lights on from the night before. I was afraid to call, to knock, to face the reality that had been rumbling toward us, despite our careful secrecy, for so long. I managed to force the door open. The smell of stale urine and feces overwhelmed me. I looked in Daddy's bedroom: He was lying beside his bed on the floor. His body was so stark, I could see the push of his rib bones against his skin. His eyes were like sunken holes and the soles of his feet were mushy, like a baby's porridge. Daddy told me, with weak lips, he'd gotten up in the night, on his way to the bathroom, and fallen down. He had been stuck there for the entire night and day, with nothing to eat or drink.

I tried to keep myself from collapsing. I told him I was going to help. I tried to move fast, but my feet and lips were as if they were in a coma. I managed to get help from the neighbor. She did not know that Daddy was struggling with AIDS; she bathed him and made him soup. I sat on the doorstep, but my complete being was in another world. Tears rushed down my cheeks like a river that has overflowed its banks.

The neighbor's daughter passed by the house and saw me. "What is wrong with your father now?" she yelled to me. I felt a sudden rush of emotion. I started breathing hard as I tried to form my words. They came out in a blur as my chest moved frantically in and out. She told me not to worry, and went in to take a look at my father to see if there was anything she could do. Daddy had told me long ago that he didn't ever want to go to the hospital, but within moments she was running out to get a taxi, racing past me without any questions asked.

I could not help but believe if I had not thought about myself and had thought about Daddy, all of this would not be happening. That was the curse of this secret: A terrible sense of responsibility, a sense that it was within my power to make my father better. Daddy was taken to the hospital, and I was sent home.

At the hospital, the nurses, who were not well educated about the virus and believed they could become infected easily, refused to touch my father. For days, he was not bathed. Often, when I went to visit him, his food was sitting untouched on his bedside table, because he was too weak to bring the food to his lips and the nurses would not feed him.

Despondent, I asked my mother for help. We found a nonprofit agency, Jamaica AIDS Support, in the phone directory, and a woman there told us about a hospice my father could go to. We called the hospice and were told by a wonderful voice on the phone that they would send over a person to come and take a look at my father. It was like Heaven on Earth. A lady came, as promised, that evening, and we both went up to the hospital to see my dad. She took one look at him and said, "You are going to be okay; we are going to take good care of you." She gave me a sense that she was interested in all that I was going through. For the first time, I felt as if I could talk, talk, talk and not be afraid of anyone or anything.

So I told her, I told her everything. I told her how I had taken care of my father on my own, I told her how I felt like killing myself, I told her how life had come to feel black and empty. She spoke to me as though she had gone through a similar experience. She told me that I was an amazing young lady and had a lot to offer to those who were not yet aware of the effects that HIV/AIDS has on families. She offered me a sliver of light at a very dark time, an opening to see that I might be able to gain something from this experience. Over time, that sliver widened, and life again began to take on meaning for me.

I was so lucky to find someone who cared. She literally saved my life. The most important thing I learned from her was this: I am not alone. In Jamaica, in the Caribbean, throughout the world, there are millions like me who first lose their childhood to a parent's illness and then lose their parent to AIDS. Worldwide, there are 15 million children who have lost at least one parent to AIDS. Eighty percent of them are in sub-Saharan Africa; the rest are scattered all over the world, including my native Jamaica. Millions of children are living in the shadow of AIDS, forced to skip school to tend to sick parents, left to scrounge for food and medicine and grow up without parental protection, guidance, and love. Most of them are cared for by already overburdened relatives. Rarely do they get any outside help. I was fortunate enough to get counseling, but in this I was an anomaly. I was so grateful for, and changed by, the help I received that I now work as a youth interventions coordinator for the National HIV AIDS prevention program in Jamaica.

I was fifteen when my father died on February 27, 2000. I will always love him, but I also feel that our secret made our wonderful relationship incomplete. I regret that. Daddy took his secret to the grave, having never spoken about AIDS to anyone, not even me. He didn't want to call attention to AIDS. I do.

the animal game; or, how i learned to take care of myself by letting others care for me

JULIA GLASS

For several months now, all my mornings have begun the same way. Just before dawn, Oliver, my five-year-old son, veers down the hallway from his bed to mine, wedges himself between me and his father, and plummets back to sleep. An hour later, he wakes and says to me, "What animal should we be today?"

I'm expected to make a suggestion, though often it's overruled. Oliver's favorites are horses, zebras, giraffes, bats, and "golden finches," though we've also been skunks, whales, squirrels, turtles, and elephants. Once we make the choice, Oliver says, "Pretend I am still in your tummy and I'm about to be born." He is quite precise, so if we're birds or reptiles, it's "Pretend I'm still in the egg and I'm about to hatch." (When he's uncertain, he'll ask, for instance, "Is an armadillo a mammal?") He curls against me, still for a moment, then stirs, struggles, and lifts his head from under the covers, blinking and smiling, a new creature greeting the unfamiliar light. I will exclaim that my baby is being born, or that I see the egg cracking— "I see a wing! I see a beak!"—and I show how happy I am.

The script is strictly programmed and tolerates only slight deviations. ("This time it takes me a long time to hatch," the actor-director may inform me.) My foal or cub or chick will "rest from being born" and then drink imaginary milk or eat an imaginary bug or worm. I pretend to clean him with my tongue or beak. If we're monkeys, I pick the nits from his head, and he reciprocates. We whinny, twitter, or trumpet; chatter like chimps. Generally, he does not choose a carnivore. Once we were owls, but when he realized that owl chicks must learn to catch and eat mice, we morphed into those favored finches. (Polar bears are fun because they shelter in snow drifts and slide on the ice, but for sustenance we can only fish, never hunt for seals. This morning we were "vegetarian sharks.")

I teach my offspring to gallop or fly or climb a tree—all while we snuggle together in bed—and then it's time for me to beg an exit, to see Alec, his ten-year-old brother, off to school. All told, the Animal Game takes five or ten minutes. It never includes his father, certainly not his brother.

A few weeks ago Oliver took the plot in a new direction. Now, every morning, we've barely begun our rest from his arduous birth when he says, "Okay, now pretend I'm growing. I'm five, six, seven . . . I'm a teenager now! Now you are having another baby." He pushes away from me a little, making space to shelter the new creature between us. He tells his tiny sibling that he will help find food for it, that he will protect it from danger: hawks if we are finches; mountain lions if we are horses; hyenas if we are zebras. He will teach it to hunt for thistle or the most delicious grass. Oliver becomes a rearing stallion, protecting us with his sharp hooves; or he is a fearsomely darting, screeching songbird, sending even the meanest raptor soaring away. I praise him for his strength and bravery. He says, "Don't worry. I will take good care of our family." Even his mother is now under his protection.

Oliver doesn't know it, but in his game he is acting out the adult transition from expecting to be cared for toward yearning to care for someone else. My generation of parents—doomed to be called the Boomers till our joints creak and any sort of booming is a thing of the past—might go down in modern history as the one that delayed this transition as long as possible, postponing parenthood to the point of recklessness, many of us fighting unnaturally hard to get there.

I can't think of anything so equally altruistic and grandiose as the longing to care for a child. It comes suddenly to some, gradually to others. Some find it after the fact—especially men who are dragged by the heels into fatherhood and then, to their dumbstruck awe, realize that they love this vacationless job. Me, I'm an agonizer. Few decisions that I make

for myself come easily. Career, mate, children, a home of my own: I've
achieved these and so many other turning points only in the nick of
time.

I gave birth to Oliver, after a surprisingly normal pregnancy, three
months shy of my forty-fifth birthday. (Alec, my older son, was five at the
time, the same age Oliver is now.) A few days later, my agent sold my first
novel. What a heady, idyllic time that was, and I knew it. Yet perhaps, deep
in my habitually agonizing self, I felt my life was too good to be true.
Something had to give.

When Oliver was four months old, I was diagnosed with a recurrence
of the breast cancer for which I'd been treated, with surgery and radiation, seven years earlier. My doctors were more shocked than I was; only
because I had obsessed over a tiny bump on my skin was the recurrence
discovered at all.

I remember sitting on the subway after getting the bad news—trying
to read a book whose dark storyline, so compelling on the ride uptown,
became unbearable on the way back down—then walking slowly from
the Union Square subway stop toward our apartment in the West Village.
I was rehearsing how I would tell this news to my mate, Dennis, when
suddenly I ran into him, two blocks from home, carrying Oliver on his
chest. "What are you doing here?" I demanded, as if it weren't logical for
them to be out and about. He told me that Oliver had been fussing, that
going out for a walk seemed the best way to calm him down.

I burst into tears. But it wasn't just the news I had to share that unleashed my grief: It was the physical confrontation, there on the corner
of Fifth Avenue and Thirteenth Street on a cold April morning, with my
responsibilities as the mother of an infant. In that moment, I discounted
Dennis's role as the very fine father he is. I looked at that bundled child
and saw him, already, as an orphan. I cried because I was scared both for
myself and for Oliver—and, of course, for his brother. I had no room for
the fear that Dennis expressed then, too, if only in his wide-eyed expression.

I remember very little about the rest of that day. Probably the first
thing I did when we got home was to remove my coat and nurse Oliver.
(My earlier cancer treatments had left me with one working breast.) No

doubt I cried my way through this quintessentially nurturing everyday act. Perhaps Dennis sat beside me, awkwardly trying to comfort me. Like many of his gender, Dennis is uncomfortable with comfort—giving or receiving. He would much rather set about, *at once,* solving the problem at hand so that comfort is moot.

Endless phone calls were made to various doctors, to set unknown wheels in motion. Dennis asked if he could make them. No, I said, I had to be the one. This wasn't strictly true, but at first I couldn't bear to let him—or anyone—help me, because to ask for help would be to admit that I was weak. How could the mother of two small children be weak? I would have to learn, though I didn't know it yet, that to accept help is both a grace and a skill. Despite years of psychotherapy—isn't that relationship a plea for help, for care?—I could not, would not, see myself as an object of care. (I suppose that's part of why I had a therapist in the first place.)

I was in high school when it suddenly became the thing to say "Take care" as you parted from friends or signed off at the end of a letter. What did we mean, these robust adolescents who had few caretaking obligations other than pets—and no desire to be cared for, except perhaps by fellow adolescents with whom we believed ourselves madly, truly in love? What we wanted most in the world was to be aggressively *independent:* no parents, no laws, no mores, no debts, no compulsory social bonds.

Years later, we would wish for dependence, for the ramparts of a family (one we'd make ourselves). But let me fine-tune the metaphor, because I picture the ideal family not as a fortress but as a tepee, a shelter of slender stakes bound tightly together at the point where their mutual leanings intersect. There's as much tension to this structure as there is shelter; without the tension, you could say, there would be no shelter. Even the smallest infant in a family is part of the supporting structure itself.

Children are yearned for, in part, for the love they give back. As they grow, that love will wax and wane, but it's part of what holds the family up. With both my babies, I had basked in the animal closeness we shared. They slept right beside me; the care they took from me they also returned.

When a baby nurses, its small hand gropes at the mother's belly or neck. It kneads, like a kitten's paw, caressing and laying claim. *Never let me go,* it says. And also, *You are mine.*

As I held Oliver on the day of my diagnosis, I felt the shocking, irresistible wish that I had not had him. If he had never been born, he would not have me to lose—nor I him. This baby had been a selfish mistake. The cancer was a cosmic shaming. It would be, I feared, the final, hardest lesson of my life, which clearly I had lived too haplessly, with too little heed for the fate of those around me.

Really, what I wanted was for him to stop needing me. I could talk to his five-year-old brother simplistically but rationally about whatever I would be facing—but there was no way that a four-month-old could let up on needing my care. There would be no bargaining with his need.

I'd heard more than one story about women diagnosed with breast cancer while pregnant, who—against medical advice—chose to delay treatment till after the child's birth. If that's not a devilish moral conundrum, I don't know what is. (With whose health, whose longevity and well-being, should you gamble?) At least I could be thankful that Oliver's birth had come before the diagnosis; how easily it could have been the other way around. I assumed it would be easy to ask, without ambivalence, for all the most aggressive (and punishing) drugs I could have. But it wasn't.

Because my recurrence was strange, fitting no medical precedents or guiding statistics, it took a dozen doctors, several diagnostic scans, and three months to finally determine that yes, I would have chemotherapy, the very treatment I'd managed to avoid when I'd first had cancer. "Bring it on," I told my oncologist.

"Listen," she warned me. "This is not going to be easy with a small child and a baby to care for. Get all the help you can." I nodded, but secretly I thought, *I can do this by myself.* That, I thought at first, was what I deserved. That was how I would prove that I was a worthy mother, that I had not let my baby down.

Foolishly, I had not yet started the difficult process of weaning Oliver.

I'd known for weeks that the systemic toxins of chemo would mean the end of viable breast milk—and that chemo was likely. But this particular intimacy, which I loved, was an antidote to my panic, and I suppose that in some parallel consciousness, I expected a magical intervention. Someone else would have the chemo for me; I had a baby to nurse! There would be two of me: the mother and the patient. How could they be one and the same? One must act as supreme caretaker, the other demand to be cared for.

We lived in close quarters back then. I worked at home in our one-bedroom apartment, writing articles and editing corporate brochures as well as working on my fiction. Four days a week, I had a babysitter, Susan, to help from ten to five. Because our place was so small—dining table and desk were one; Dennis and I slept on a bed in the living room—she often took Oliver out for the day. Dennis, a photographer with a one-man studio, kept long hours, rarely getting home before seven in the evening, often working till nine or ten—as well as most weekends.

Weaning Oliver, in under two weeks, was sheer hell. He would not accept a bottle while held against my chest. At first, he would protest even if I was in the apartment while Dennis or Susan tried to feed him. The bedtime feeding was the worst. I would retreat to the tiny kitchen or aimlessly, heartlessly leave the apartment while Oliver wrestled in his father's arms, sometimes crying himself to sleep.

Not until the last possible moment did I tell my friends I'd be having the chemo. Once I did, a few of them offered to pitch in by taking Alec now and then, for an evening or a weekend afternoon. The poignant truth, however, was that I didn't need much help with Alec. I was shocked to discover, when I stood back, that he no longer required much physical aid, the kind that requires strength, energy, and the ample patience of the hale and hardy. He needed me to walk him places, hold his hand while crossing the street, read to him, talk with him, turn out his lights and kiss him good night—but he did not need to be lifted, carried, bathed, or fed by me. He was filled with the radiant confidence of having started kindergarten: "real school," as he so proudly called it.

"Thank you," I'd say to my kind friends, "but Alec isn't really the one I'll need help with." Did I ask outright for help with Oliver? No. These friends had toddlers and babies of their own; how could they take on another?

"Isn't your mother coming down to help?" some would ask. I was regularly in touch with my mother, who lived in Massachusetts. When I told her about the recurrence, she said, almost at once, "I know you're going to get through this, and you're going to live to see your boys through college. I know it. I have a sense for these things." *No, you don't! No one does!* I wanted to yell. She also said, and I had to agree, that it would probably not be a good idea for her to come to New York.

The most intense memories I have of being nursed through illness are those of my mother's comforts and remedies whenever I had a bad cold as a child: her hand on my head to search for fever, the hot water bottle (wrapped in a hand towel so it wouldn't scald), the ice-cold silvery Vicks she'd spread on my chest, the hot toddy she'd make with orange juice, lemon, and honey (did she add a dash of my father's bourbon?). It always arrived at my bedside in the same Creamsicle lusterware mug. She'd carry it up to my room and hold the hot mug while I sipped the sweet-and-sour elixir, letting its steam clear my nose.

As adults, however, my mother and I have had a hard time getting along when the going gets tough. Facing the same crisis brings out the worst in both of us—probably the identical worst, thanks to the orchestration of our genes. So I did not feel offended by her suggesting that she stay away. I should say, too, that the distance she kept was necessary not just for our harmony but for her sanity. She had already lost another grown daughter, my little sister, who'd taken her own life eight years before. To see the physical evidence of my potential early demise as well—really now, how could she suffer that?

And why should she, or anyone other than me, experience any pointless suffering? A certain solitude seemed perfectly apt. I was the one who'd cope with the effects of the chemo, so I could cope with the coping, too.

But this didn't mean I wasn't scared—and maudlin at times. I found myself having melodramatic visions as I waited for the first bout of treatment: I saw myself gaunt and jaundiced, skin drooping off atrophied muscles; vomiting, succumbing to a deadly opportunistic infection. I saw myself in a hospital gown. *But wait!* I'd think. These visions conflicted, perplexingly, with the image I had of myself standing fast as a mother, continuing to shop and cook, read stories, sing lullabies—and work. One thing I knew for certain: When a household comprises two self-employed people with modest incomes, no one gets time off for a medical crisis. We have the stingiest employers of all. (Maternity leave? I was proofreading magazine galleys the day I got home from having Alec; Oliver, in his first months, I'd breast-fed on my lap while typing revisions to my first novel.)

All of a sudden, I received a spate of gifts: bath accessories (the standout was a jar of gray granules called Tired Old Ass), murder mysteries, boxes of candy, nightgowns, and fluffy socks. Did anyone think that my life could really slow down enough for leisurely baths and days spent lounging in lingerie? And in the bodily onslaught to come, I needed Albert Schweitzer, not Fanny Farmer. (Yes, the famously nauseating agents now came with a counterpunch of three antinausea drugs, whose own side effects were to be palliated in turn by an everyday laxative. I'd be able to eat, but honestly . . . chocolate-covered cherries?) And here's a riddle I'd love to have answered: Why in the world would anyone want to read about murder when death is the very thing they are hoping to cheat?

And yet, as scornful as I felt about some of these gifts, I was touched. They drew from within me the undeniable desire, strong as an undertow, to lie down and be cared for, to put my life as a mother on hold. How I wanted to be, though I couldn't have confessed this to anyone, the baby. Already, just from the anxiety, fear, and pangs of sheer hopelessness, I felt at times disabled. I wanted the grown-up equivalent of being swaddled and sung to, held without words. A baby chimp, a bird in a nest, a joey in her mother's furry pouch. And the ordeal—the physical part—had yet to begin.

Chemotherapy is, in some ways, anticlimactic. The moment it begins is surreal and terrifying: if you let yourself think about the indiscriminately destructive way in which this medicine will go to work, the friendly fire you are about to unleash on your body along with the special ops, it feels like you're flirting with death. (Well, you already were.) But then it becomes more like a new career. The lists of tasks, tests, pills, appointments, precautions, and prohibitions were so formidable that I bought a new calendar just to keep track of them all. Practically speaking, subjecting yourself to chemotherapy is as bureaucratic as doing your taxes or taking out a mortgage. You're so busy following the rules that you forget to anticipate the side effects you feared so much when you first got the news you'd be joining this club.

As for the drugs themselves, the way they affect you varies greatly from one to the next. I would have six months of treatment—three of one type, three of another—to be given one day out of every three weeks. With all the blood tests, the waiting for this and that, the drugs given in advance to reduce side effects and prevent allergic reactions, never mind the drawn-out intravenous administration of the big guns themselves (which often took over an hour), each session generally lasted the entire day. Dennis insisted on being with me through the first of these days (there would be eight altogether). I acquiesced, though I told him that during subsequent treatments I wanted him either to work or, if our sitter was off, to be with the kids. To be with me when I was surrounded by professionals would be a waste of time. At the clinic, I pointed out patients who appeared to be there solo. "See?" I said. "If they can go it alone, so can I."

I do remember the opening salvo, the first dose winding its way from a plastic pouch down into my arm. *I have agreed to let myself be poisoned,* I thought with horror and wonder. *This is for my children,* I'd sometimes think during later treatments or when they made me feel particularly ill. I began to understand how people decide to turn down treatment even if it means life will be shorter.

My oncologist, a warm, outspoken woman, would make her way among the patients to see how we were doing. She would hug us. I remember how startling this was, the first time she did it. She was giving us permission to acknowledge how fragile we felt. I was touched—and also embarrassed.

Dennis's youngest sister, an energetic law student in her twenties, came out from Montana for two weeks. The idea was that Jane would help out while doing a bit of sightseeing and visiting with her nephews. She went with me to my second treatment. By then I had lost my hair.

I was supposed to steer clear of the sun and stay out of crowds. (In August. In New York City.) One evening Dennis and Jane took the boys to an outdoor movie—the forbidden crowd scene. I said I was fine staying home. I would rest. I sat around feeling sorry for myself. So many old consolations—pasta, chocolate, rich books, weepy movies on the VCR—made me miserable now.

Another night, I took Jane out for a Greek meal, determined that I would act normal. ("Smile if it kills you," my mother used to scold, quoting her staunch German mother.) "I'm okay. This is delicious!" I kept saying over the meal. This was half true. It tasted like a memory of delicious, like this would be delicious *if*.

When Jane went back west, Dennis grumbled that she had probably created more work for us than she had given help. I argued that this wasn't so. I didn't say what I knew: that if her visit had been extra work, it was only because I had refused to let her help "too much"—wash too many dishes, hold Oliver too often. A combination of guilt and courtesy (*She's our guest!*) held me back from simply letting go.

My datebook from August 2001 is a welter of scrawled obligations, normal enough at a glance. But a typical day might read, *Bloods 10:30/Bone scan 1:00/Alec—playdate with Emma 3:00/bill JPMorgan for client brochure/ buy kindergarten supplies.* One day is marked over in urgent black letters *NADIR POINT.* This was the midpoint between every two chemo sessions when my immune system was at its lowest ebb, most vulnerable to a multitude of germs and infections. I was to live as if I were touring in a Third World country: eat no raw fruit or vegetables whatsoever, wash hands often, steer clear of anyone who seemed vaguely ill, avoid mosquito bites.

People told me I looked great. I did not lose or gain weight. I tied festive scarves around my head. I did not stop going to parties. I felt like one of those apples whose shiny, firm appearance conceals a mealy, brown interior. Beneath the skin, it's little more than a massive bruise.

· · ·

Our sitter, Susan, had been working for us only a month or so when I found out about the recurrence. She was a steady, dependable young woman with a child older than both of mine. Her ease and tenderness with Oliver were ample, but she was businesslike and quiet around me and Dennis. There was no chitchat, nor did she ever watch TV. If she and I shared the apartment while Oliver napped, she'd read a magazine. Susan had shown concern and sympathy when she heard about the cancer, but she did not pry. She was (still is) one of those rare souls who lives well with silence.

At first, once the treatment started, I felt awkward around her—but then her quiet steadiness steadied me as well. Dennis would make every effort to stay home until she arrived at ten each morning, but he could rarely make it back home earlier than seven; because Susan had to be home to meet her daughter after school, she could never stay later than five. I came to dread the margin of time between Susan's departure and Dennis's return. Feeling ill, weak, and dismayed, I had two children on my hands who needed feeding, bathing, and entertaining in different, often conflicting ways. Oliver would be wide awake, wanting to be held and jiggled. In previous months, we'd had a ritual of dancing to lively music while I held him on my hip. I could no longer dance without becoming dizzy. Alec would want to hear a story or play with his trains. I could get down on the floor to lay tracks, but getting up again was torture.

The minute Dennis came in the door, I would snap like an overextended elastic. And I was, no help to Dennis, almost always more cranky than grateful. Since there was no real privacy in our small home, Alec would see me angry or in tears. I would blame it on my "sickness" or the "medicine," both of which he grasped in the broadest of terms.

But really, I ought to have placed the blame on my pride.

The turning point may have been a searingly hot day that August when I was almost too weak to carry Oliver up the stairs of our building. Or it may have been the departure of my sister-in-law, when I realized how little I'd taken advantage of her willing presence. But certainly by that September 11—when suddenly I was far, *far* from the neediest person around—and definitely by the next week, when Alec broke his leg in school, I understood something achingly, pathetically obvious. Accepting help, even asking for it, was not about me. To hell with the notion that I didn't "deserve" the care of others. Alec and Oliver deserved that care—theirs, yes, but also mine. My care was but an extension of theirs. We were the stakes of that tepee; our stability was a matter of mutual dependence.

A friend of mine who is uneasy around small children but cooks like a pro offered to make Dennis and me several compact dinners, bring them over, and put them in our freezer. I felt myself wanting to tell her no, that was too much to ask, not necessary, but I said, "Yes. Thank you! That would be wonderful." And it was. I remember the look of loving satisfaction on Lindsay's face when she arrived with a bag of neatly foil-wrapped packages. She made us risotto, orzo, pearl couscous, each dish cooked with a different assortment of vegetables. The mere presence of these dinners in the freezer was soothing, even before we'd take them out and, on our most defeated nights, heat them in the oven and consume their rich, starchy, buttery comfort—comfort we were both very glad I'd accepted.

Another friend, Lucy, whose previous offers of help I'd turned down with one excuse after another, persisted. One day she said, "Why don't you just pick one evening a week, and I'll come over and do whatever you need me to do until Dennis comes home? Let me do *something*." She sounded just a little, and justifiably, exasperated. Get over it, she was telling me. Yes, I said again. So once a week she'd arrive straight from work, with groceries—whatever I felt I could eat that night—and she'd chat and read with Alec and put him to bed while I bathed Oliver and gave him the bottle he had finally learned to accept without protest. Then Lucy would make me sit down while she cooked me dinner, and we would eat together. We'd watch a movie or talk. Dennis could stay late at his studio with a clear conscience, and when he came home, she'd leave. Or she'd hang around. Listening to her light conversation with Dennis, I realized he needed this, too: the company of someone, at the end of his day, who wasn't wearing a mantle of gravestone granite.

I decided that I would make sure someone accompanied me to all my remaining treatments. I would ask a different friend each time. I would stop feeling silly because other patients were there alone. "So what hap-

pens?" my friends would ask, a little awestruck but always, to my surprise,
flattered. "Mainly a lot of sitting around," I'd say. "Bring something to read.
Something long."

The drug I received for the last three months of treatment required
a hit of tranquilizer that left me dazed yet absurdly ingratiating. The first
time I received it, I tried to converse politely with my companion and
heard myself sounding like a bonehead. The next time, I let myself fall
asleep. I remember coming to, briefly, and smiling at my friend Lindsay
(the fine cook), who looked up from her book before I drifted off again.
Perhaps I snored, or drooled, while she sat there beside me. Perhaps it
was the dullest day of her week—or the most oddly relaxing. And me—
gradually I was learning to live, while in the company of others, with
unapologetic silence.

One of my oldest, most outgoing friends, a man who has had a lot
of experience with illness in his own life, scrutinized the complex results
of that day's blood tests. These tests were administered weekly and on the
morning before each treatment. Habitually, I accepted the printout from
the lab but never asked what the columns of numbers signified. "This is
excellent news," my outgoing friend said, pointing to one of the numbers.
"And this, this is very impressive, the perfect level to be at!" The compli-
ments he paid my blood cheered me up, even lent me a sense of modest
accomplishment. He also went out of his way to befriend "our" nurse
that day. The two of them exchanged wry jokes about drawing blood and
taking urine samples. My friend touched me on the arm (the one not
connected to pouches of poison), commenting heartily and loudly, "Most
people don't realize this, but a good phlebotomist is worth her weight in
gold." After all I'd been through, all the times my veins had been prodded,
squeezed, and punctured, I had to agree. This remains one of the warmer,
loonier moments I remember from that entire six months.

Wit, I came to realize, is a precious and essential kind of care when
one is ill—not jokes; just the weird new perspective of someone who
stands on the outside yet loves you and wants to see you well and happy.
Dennis had recently spotted bicycle messengers zipping around town with
LED strips mounted behind them, clever advertising space for all manner
of local commerce, from ministorage to livery cabs. My bald head, he sug-

gested, might be useful to sell as an advertising opportunity. We decided I
could wear an LED headband with a revolving commercial similar to the
strip of headlines that orbits the center of Times Square. "How about," I
suggested, thinking of all the pharmaceutical ads lately proliferating on TV,
"'Adriamycin! Ask your doctor if it's right for you.'"

The side effects of my various drugs were colorful and eclectic. The
third drug I took was, I liked to say back then, a pact with the devil. Gone
were the digestive ailments and the gum sores, but quick to take their
place was a severe, migratory bone pain that kept me up for hours at night.
It felt like a series of deep-seated charley-horse cramps, occurring now
in my hip, now in my shoulder, perhaps in my left shin and right thigh at
once. Shifting position in bed made no difference, for the pain had nothing to do with muscles or tendons, though that's exactly what it felt like.

Oliver still woke for a feeding in the middle of the night. On those
nights when I was enduring this pain, I was already awake myself, but the
relentless cramping made it impossible to hold Oliver steadily enough to
give him a bottle. So Dennis would rise, too, and we'd sit in bed, next to
each other, awake for different reasons. "This really, really, really hurts," I'd
gasp.

"I wish there was something I could do," Dennis would answer quietly. He didn't touch me; the mere idea of being touched was horrendous
to me.

What I didn't tell him, but should have, was that he was doing something just by being awake with me. I began to understand that taking care
of someone doesn't always mean doing something for that person; there
isn't always a hot toddy or a water bottle or an ointment to soothe. Being
is just as important as doing. Being awake. Being present in the next chair.
Being funny. Being smart in a surprising, useful way. Being sympathetically perplexed. Being a mirror for the expression of pain.

About a week after September 11, Lucy and I were sitting together eating the pasta she'd made the two of us for dinner. We'd been through our
evening routine with the boys and I assumed they were long asleep.

Lucy and I were talking about how embarrassed we were to know so little about the part of the world on which Americans were now intently focused. Pakistan had just been strong-armed into acting as an emissary to the Taliban, and we were wondering if anything would come of this desperate overture.

Suddenly Alec entered the room and asked what we were discussing.

"Alec, go back to bed," I said.

"I will go back to bed," he declared, "if you tell me one thing you were talking about. One thing."

I sighed. "Well, we were saying that the people who know where Osama bin Laden is hiding won't tell us where he is. They're protecting him." (Alec, like every other five-year-old in Lower Manhattan, knew all about the manhunt by now.)

His face brightened. "I have an idea. We should hypnotize the guys who are the protectors, and then they will tell us where Osama bin Laden is, and then the police will turn him into a good guy."

Lucy and I laughed with approval. "Honey, that's a brilliant idea," I said. "I bet they never thought of hypnosis. But now you need to go to bed." And without further protest, he did, my little statesman. Like his father, he wanted to help solve the problem at the root of so much grief. Perhaps he'd even lain awake that week, wondering how he could help catch the felon.

Lucy turned to me and said, "Quick! Let's e-mail the CIA!"

"Here's the plan," I said. "We send the Pakistanis back to Kabul. We give them—how big is the Taliban?—a hundred pocket watches. And then there they are, waving those watches: 'You are getting sleeeeepier and sleeeeepier, you are getting very, very sleepy. . . .' You know, it just might work."

We laughed so hard that, for a minute, I felt cured of so many things. Oh, the world was a cruel, crazy, chaotic place all right, about to see much more violence unleashed (would the president have defended our invasions as comparable to chemotherapy, side effects all for the good of the greater body?). But I had a family, and friends, to help me retain the best of myself, my humor and hope, my fortitude.

. . .

When the weather turned fierce, Lindsay—a seamstress as well as a cook—made me four slinky velvet caps with tassels. I could wear them all day, indoors and out. They made me look like a tall, jaunty elf. One was black, one dusty teal, one leopard, one a neon shade of tangerine. The tassels, which swung as I walked along, tickled the side of my neck.

Pushed by the drugs, I was catapulted rudely, *splat,* into menopause. I got through the holidays learning not to hide from family cameras just because I had no eyebrows or lashes (or just because I was suddenly breaking out in rivulets of unprovoked perspiration). I looked . . . sleek, perhaps. People told me how beautiful my skin had become. "It's the not drinking," I'd quip. Or, in select company, "It's finally losing the acne, along with ovulation."

Dennis and I concocted our 2002 New Year's card by photographing the back of my naked head, my bright orange elf cap pushed up on top, with the words *Happy New Year* projected right onto my rosy scalp. It was colorful and wry, such a perfect expression of how bleak we felt about the bad year behind us (and, as it turned out, everyone else) and yet how our hope and humor endured. We usually argue over the making of the annual card, but this time we were in cahoots. "You know what? This is sick!" we said at one point. But sick, that's what we'd been dealing with for months. We knew from sick.

I was often sore, often cranky, often in spiritual wilt. By this point, so was Dennis. Sometimes I'd know, just from looking at him, that he'd had enough, that his well of mercy was running dry. This did not help, because—though I'd never say so—I needed him to be a saint. (*That's your job—saint!* I wanted to yell. *Just do your job!*) But the demands of my children's schedules, the knowledge that I was capable of working and so I would, the drive to "be myself"—all kept me going until, one day in January, the chemotherapy came to an end. Over, just like that.

I began to feel better. And regrow hair. And look forward to spring. And eat like a normal, hungry person. And carry Oliver on my chest again. And go running.

And miss the extra attentions of my friends, their company and their concern. Why in the world had I not seized on their caretaking from the very start? All of a sudden, I became fixated on the rearview mirror, nostalgic for the invalid state I had never quite achieved. I had never, after all, been bedridden, checked into the hospital, called an ambulance. I'd had one close call, in which a fleck of dirt under a thumbnail—lodged there while I was shelling lima beans—caused an alarming infection that spread all the way to my elbow. But that was the most dramatic moment in six months of what I'd once assumed would be a time of unrelenting pain, mourning, solemnity, even stasis. (Leave it to me to face the gravest danger under such ludicrous circumstances. Once I'd been brought back from the brink of gangrene, did the nurses ever have a field day with me. "If it isn't the lima-bean girl!" I'd be greeted at reception. Or "Didn't anyone ever tell you they come in cans?" And "You, like, eat them by *choice*?")

Cancer patients often feel letdown, not relief, when treatment ends. What remains, once the "good fight" is over? "Getting back to life!" says the person who's never had cancer. *Waiting for the next fight,* the rest of us can't help thinking. My letdown—textbook—took the form of self-pity. "I never got to just lie down and just get taken care of!" I complained to Dennis. He shot me a look of rue and exasperation. As if I hadn't shaken up his life but good.

After the letdown came, also textbook, the flood of gratitude. Who was I fooling? Of course I'd been "taken care of," and richly. By Susan, our sitter, who'd behaved as if everything were normal—and, by doing so, helped make life as normal as it could possibly be for those who mattered most: my sons. By Dennis, who'd twisted his schedule into a pretzel . . . along with his psyche, if simply by never (well, almost never) giving in to panic or rage. By my friends, who shared their many and various talents, who made themselves available, who put up with my vain pretense that really, I was fine coping all by myself.

Finally, too, I understood that I had begun to learn to take care of myself—or, rather, to learn that taking care of myself required being cared for by others at the very same time. This calls for a balancing of humility and pride that may come naturally to many, but not to me. Only by facing what I owed others as well as myself did I come to my senses.

· · ·

Five years have passed without another crisis of health in our family. Last year we moved to another state so that we could have a home with more than one bedroom and live closer to my aging parents ... whom I may one day need to care for whether they like the idea or not. (Would it surprise you to know they do not?) In sacrifice to these practical concerns, Dennis has given up, at least temporarily, a profession that worked well for him even if it worked him too hard. For the past year, he has been doing something that few men could do with such grace: He is letting me support the family. He is now the primary hands-on caretaker, the one who packs school lunches and takes the boys to their sports, oversees their playdates. With the help of his own sharp wit, he, too, has embraced the humility of being cared for. This arrangement won't last forever, we both know, but that doesn't make it any easier.

I am reminded of the Animal Game, Oliver's wishing first to be the baby, then the protector; then, next morning, the baby all over again. If we're fortunate, we trade these roles back and forth— dependence and dependability, helplessness and helpfulness; odd mixtures of both—in ever more complicated relays, all our lives, to the very end. Grown children care for parents, wives for husbands, brothers for sisters, friends for friends. Pretend I am just being born, we say when we are struck down by illness. Pretend I am resting because it was hard. Feed me. Clean me. Hold me close. Take care of me—and then, let me take care of you.

contributors

JULIA ALVAREZ is the author of several novels, including *Saving the World, How the Garcia Girls Lost Their Accents,* and *In the Time of the Butterflies,* as well as a book of essays, *Something to Declare,* and several poetry books, among them, *The Woman I Kept to Myself.* She has also written for children and young adults, most recently *Before We Were Free* and *finding miracles.* She is a writer-in-residence at Middlebury College, and with her husband, Bill Eichner, has established Alta Gracia, a sustainable-farm-literary project in her native Dominican Republic, where her elderly parents now live.

NELL CASEY is the editor of the national bestseller *Unholy Ghost: Writers on Depression.* Her writing has appeared in the *New York Times,* Slate, Salon, *Elle, Cookie, Self,* and *Fitness,* among other publications. She lives in Brooklyn with her husband and son.

ELEANOR COONEY is the author of *Death in Slow Motion* (HarperCollins, 2004), which grew out of the *Harper's* magazine article of the same name. She's the coauthor of three novels set in T'ang dynasty China, and is at work on a literary thriller set in the Royal College of Surgeons in London. She has written articles for *Mother Jones* magazine, including "The Way It Was" (Sept./Oct. 2004) about pre-*Roe* abortion. She's expanding the article into a book that explores, among many other things, what various great authors have written about illegal abortion. She lives in Mendocino, California. Contact her through: www.deathinslowmotion.com.

AMANDA FORTINI is a regular Slate contributor. She has also written for the *New York Times Book Review,* the *New York Times Magazine, I.D.,* the *Forward,* and *New York* magazine, among other publications. She lives in Los Angeles.

JULIA GLASS is the author of two novels: *Three Junes,* which won the 2002 National Book Award for Fiction, and *The Whole World Over.* She has been honored with grants and fellowships from the National Endowment for the Arts, the New York Foundation for the Arts, and the Radcliffe Institute for Advanced Study. For her short fiction, she has won several awards, including the Tobias Wolff Award and the Pirate's Alley Faulkner Society Medal for Best Novella. Her essay "I Have a Crush on Ted Geisel" was published in *Kiss Tomorrow Hello: Notes from the Midlife Underground by Twenty-Five Women over Forty,* edited by Kim Barnes and Claire Davis. She lives with her family in Massachusetts.

JEROME E. GROOPMAN, M.D., holds the Dina and Raphael Re-canti Chair of Medicine at the Harvard Medical School and is chief of experimental medicine at the Beth Israel Deaconess Medical Center. He received his B.A. from Columbia College summa cum laude and his M.D. from Columbia College of Physicians and Surgeons in New York. He served his internship and residency in internal medicine at the Massachu-setts General Hospital, and his specialty fellowships in hematology and oncology at the University of California, Los Angeles, and the Children's Hospital/Sidney Farber Cancer Center, Harvard Medical School in Bos-ton. He serves on many scientific editorial boards and has published more than 150 scientific articles. In 2000, he was elected to the Institute of Medicine of the National Academy of Sciences.

Dr. Groopman has authored numerous editorials on policy issues in the *New Republic,* the *Washington Post,* and the *New York Times.* His first popular book, *The Measure of Our Days,* published in October 1997, ex-plores the spiritual lives of patients with serious illness. This was the ba-sis for the ABC television series *Gideon's Crossing.* In 1998, he became a staff writer in medicine and biology at the *New Yorker* magazine. His next book, entitled *Second Opinions,* was published in February 2000, and his third book, *The Anatomy of Hope,* was released in 2004 and was a *New York Times* bestseller. His most recent book, *How Doctors Think,* published in March 2007, explores how physicians arrive at the correct diagnosis and treatment, and why they may not.

ANN HARLEMAN is the author of two short-story collections—*Happiness,* which won the Iowa Short Fiction Award, and *Thoreau's Laundry*—and two novels, *Bitter Lake* and *The Year She Disappeared.* Among her awards are Guggenheim and Rockefeller fellowships, three Rhode Island States Arts Council fellowships, the Berlin Prize in Literature, the PEN Syndicated Fiction Award, the O. Henry Award, and a Rona Jaffe Writer's Award.

In an earlier life, having been the first woman to receive a Ph.D. in linguistics from Princeton, Harleman lived and worked behind the Iron Curtain. Now happily teaching fiction writing to visual artists, she is on the faculties of Brown University and the Rhode Island School of Design. She can be reached through her website, www.annharleman.com.

ANN HOOD is the author of seven novels, including *Somewhere off the Coast of Maine* and, most recently, *The Knitting Circle;* a collection of short stories, *An Ornithologist's Guide to Life;* and a memoir, *Do Not Go Gentle: My Search for Miracles in a Cynical Time.* Her essays and stories have appeared in many publications, including the *New York Times,* the *Paris Review, Glimmer Train, Tin House,* and *Ploughshares.* She has twice won a Pushcart Prize as well as a Best American Spiritual Writing Award and the Paul Bowles Prize for Short Fiction. She lives in Providence, Rhode Island.

ANNE LANDSMAN is the author of *The Rowing Lesson* and *The Devil's Chimney.* Her writing has also appeared in the *Washington Post,* the *American Poetry Review, Poets and Writers, The Believer,* and *Bomb* and she has an essay in the anthology *The Honeymoon's Over.*

ED BOK LEE is the author of *Real Karaoke People,* winner of the PEN/ Beyond Margins Award and the Members' Choice Asian American Literary Award. He's studied Russian and central Asian languages and literatures at the Universities of California at Berkeley, Minnesota, Kazakh State, Almaty, and holds an MFA from Brown University. Various other awards for his writing include support from the Jerome Foundation and the National Endowment for the Arts.

SUSAN LEHMAN is the director of communications and strategy for the Brennan Center for Justice, a think tank and public-interest law firm. She is the author, with Edward W. Hayes, of *Mouthpiece: My Life in—and Just Outside—the Law,* with an introduction by Tom Wolfe (Doubleday). Formerly an editor at *Talk* magazine, Salon, and Penguin Books, Lehman has also written about law, crime, travel, and entertainment for a range of publications including the *New York Times,* the *Atlantic Monthly,* the *New Yorker, GQ, Vogue, Glamour,* and the late *SPY* magazine. She is a former criminal defense lawyer and lives in New York with her children.

SAM LIPSYTE's most recent novel is *Home Land,* a *New York Times* Notable Book for 2005 and winner of the Believer Book Award. He is also the author of *The Subject Steve* and *Venus Drive.* His work has appeared in *The Quarterly, Open City, N+1,* Slate, *McSweeney's, Esquire, Bookforum,* the *New York Times,* and *Playboy,* among other places. He teaches at Columbia University.

STAN MACK is a reporter-cartoonist who pioneered a documentary style of cartooning with his notorious New York comic strip *Stan Mack's Real Life Funnies,* which ran in the *Village Voice* for twenty years. His *Ad-Week* magazine comic strip, *Stan Mack's Outtakes,* covered the New York media scene for a decade. He has used his trademark style in newspapers, magazines, and books. His latest book, from which the essay in this collection is excerpted, is *Janet & Me: An Illustrated Story of Love and Loss.* He has created two graphic histories, *The Story of the Jews: A 4,000 Year Adventure* and *Stan Mack's Real Life Revolution.* He is the coauthor, with his late partner, Janet Bode, of several young adult nonfiction books including *Heartbreak and Roses, Hard Time,* and *For Better, for Worse.* He has also created children's picture books, including the bestselling *10 Bears in My Bed.*

He is currently working on a series of graphic historical novels for teens. A graduate of the Rhode Island School of Design, Mack is a former art director of the *New York Times Magazine.*

FRANK McCOURT, acclaimed memoirist and Pulitzer Prize winner, was born in New York City and raised in Limerick, Ireland, in the 1930s and 1940s. At the age of nineteen, McCourt returned to the United States. After graduating from New York University's School of Education, he found a brilliant career as a New York public high school teacher.

In September 1996, after he had retired from teaching, McCourt's memoir of his childhood, *Angela's Ashes,* was published by Scribner. It quickly rose to the top of the hardcover bestseller lists, remaining on the *New York Times* list for 117 weeks. It was also selected as the number one nonfiction book of the year by *Time* and *Newsweek.*

Angela's Ashes won many awards, including the Pulitzer Prize, the National Book Critics' Circle Award, the ABBY Award, and the *Los Angeles Times* Book Award. With the release of the film version of *Angela's Ashes,* directed by Alan Parker, the paperback edition also achieved bestseller status.

In September 1999, McCourt published the follow-up to *Angela's Ashes,* titled *'Tis: A Memoir,* which hit the *New York Times* bestseller list at number one, as did the paperback edition. *'Tis* received the New York Society Library Award and Italy's Riccardo Bacchelli Award.

November 2005 saw the publication of *Teacher Man* and its immediate jump to number one on the *New York Times* bestseller list. In 2007, Scribner will publish *Angela and the Baby Jesus,* a children's Christmas story.

McCourt's acclaimed musical revue, *The Irish and How They Got That Way,* ran for more than a year at the Irish Repertory Theatre in New York. And the two-man play *A Couple of Blaguards* continues to be produced throughout the United States, Canada, and Australia.

McCourt has one daughter, Maggie, and three grandchildren: Chiara, Frankie, and Jack. He frequently lectures, mainly at universities across the country. He is also collaborating with composer David Amram on a New York City–inspired mass called *Missa Manhattan.* He lives with his wife, Ellen, and dog, Rory, in Connecticut and New York City.

KERREL MCKAY is a twenty-two-year-old Jamaican, who cofounded Claudia Williams Life Center in 2000, a center for young people to access information about HIV/AIDS and other sexual reproductive health services and a place where those infected and affected can go to get care and support. She then moved on to advocacy on an international stage, where she represented UNICEF at various meetings and conferences around the world, including Brazil, Thailand, Africa, and France. Soon after, she began interviewing young people for the UNICEF Voices of the Youth program. She is a teacher by profession but to date is employed with the Ministry of Health in Kingston, Jamaica, as the youth interventions coordinator in the National HIV/AIDS Program.

JUSTINE PICARDIE is a writer who lives in London with her husband and two sons. Her books include *If the Spirit Moves You,* a memoir about the death of her sister, and *My Mother's Wedding Dress.* Her latest novel, *Daphne,* will be published by Bloomsbury.

HELEN SCHULMAN is the author of the novels *A Day at the Beach, P.S., The Revisionist,* and *Out of Time,* and the short-story collection *Not a Free Show. P.S.* was also made into a feature film starring Laura Linney. She co-edited, along with Jill Bialosky, the anthology *Wanting a Child.* Her fiction and nonfiction have appeared in such places as *Vanity Fair, Time, Vogue, GQ,* the *New York Times Book Review,* and the *Paris Review.* She is presently the fiction coordinator at the writing program at the New School.

SCOT SEA lives with his wife and daughter in Tucson, Arizona.

ANDREW SOLOMON is the author of *The Irony Tower: Soviet Artists in a Time of Glasnost* (Knopf, 1991) and *A Stone Boat* (Faber, 1994), which was a runner-up for the *Los Angeles Times* First Fiction prize and was a national bestseller; it has now been published in five languages. His most recent book, *The Noonday Demon: An Atlas of Depression,* has won fourteen national awards, including the 2001 National Book Award, and is being published in twenty-two languages. He is a regular contributor to numerous publications, including the *New York Times,* the *New Yorker,* and *Artfo-*

rum, and is currently writing a book, to be published in 2008 by Scribner called *A Dozen Kinds of Love: Raising Traumatic Children,* which deals with how families accommodate children who are deaf, who are autistic, who are prodigies, who have committed crimes, and so on, for which he has been awarded residencies at Yaddo, MacDowell, and the Rockefeller Foundation Bellagio. He is also working on a comic novel. He maintains residences in London and New York and is a dual national.

ABIGAIL THOMAS's most recent book is *A Three Dog Life* (2006), a memoir covering the five years after an accident caused her husband traumatic brain injury. She lives in Woodstock, New York, and is the author of *Safekeeping,* also a memoir, and three books of fiction—*Herb's Pajamas, An Actual Life,* and *Getting Over Tom.* Her husband died in January 2007.

STEPHEN YADZINSKI's writing has appeared in the *New York Times Magazine.* He is also a photo illustrator and an artist. He lives with his wife and son in Santa Fe, New Mexico. He can be reached at http://yadzinski.us.

acknowledgments

There are many people to whom I am grateful for their advice and support: Stacy Abramson, Ginia Bellafante, Tessa Blake, Seth Romse, Bliss Broyard, Capricia Buchanan, Jenny Carchman, Clare Casey, Connie Casey, John Casey, Julia Casey, Maud Casey, Ros Casey, Ernie Drucker, Jeri Drucker, Jesse Eisinger, Sarah Ellison, Virginia Heffernan, Tovi Kratovil, Lori Leibovich, Carol Levine of the United Hospital Fund, Josh Shenk, Lorraine Tobias, Harold Varmus, Shannon Worrell, Joey Xanders.

To my mother, Jane Barnes, who taught me everything I know about caring.

To Kim Witherspoon and Alexis Hurley for making it happen.

To my editors, Alison Callahan and Jeanette Perez.

To Jesse and Hank Drucker, reasons for being.

And to the contributors, without whom this book would not exist.

permissions

EDITED BY NELL CASEY

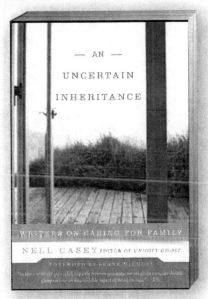

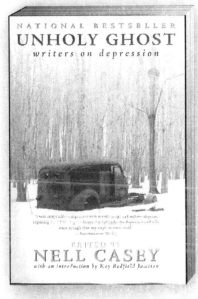

AN UNCERTAIN INHERITANCE
Writers on Caring for Family

ISBN 978-0-06-087531-2 (paperback)

"These essays about caring for gravely
ill parents, partners, even children,
meet a real need.... Though wrenching,
the stories provide solace and practical
advice." — People

"A godsend for many readers."
— Newsday

"Honest...[a] remarkably wide spectrum
of experiences is covered."
— New York Times Book Review

UNHOLY GHOST
Writers on Depression

ISBN 978-0-06-000782-9 (paperback)

"These essays address depression with
notable sanity and stylistic elegance,
exploring the debilitating conditions
that fall under the depression umbrella
more strongly than any single memoir
could." — Entertainment Weekly

"As a whole, the collection is a valuable
contribution to the field of depression
studies, and will lend some insight and
cheer to those struggling with this little-
understood condition."
— Publishers Weekly

"The quality of the essays in Unholy
Ghost is outstanding." — Newsday

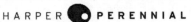

CPSIA information can be obtained at www.ICGtesting.com
Printed in the USA
LVOW08s1228190116

471264LV00011B/65/P